End-of-Life Nursing Care

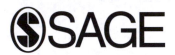

End-of-Life Nursing Care

a guide for best practice

Joanna De Souza and Annie Pettifer

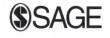

Los Angeles | London | New Delhi
Singapore | Washington DC

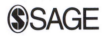

Los Angeles | London | New Delhi
Singapore | Washington DC

SAGE Publications Ltd
1 Oliver's Yard
55 City Road
London EC1Y 1SP

SAGE Publications Inc.
2455 Teller Road
Thousand Oaks, California 91320

SAGE Publications India Pvt Ltd
B 1/I 1 Mohan Cooperative Industrial Area
Mathura Road
New Delhi 110 044

SAGE Publications Asia-Pacific Pte Ltd
3 Church Street
#10-04 Samsung Hub
Singapore 049483

Editor: Susan Worsey
Assistant Editor: Emma Milman
Production editor: Katie Forsythe
Proofreader: Bryan Campbell
Marketing manager: Tamara Navaratnam
Cover design: Jennifer Crisp
Typeset by: C&M Digitals (P) Ltd, Chennai, India
Printed by: MPG Books Group, Bodmin, Cornwall

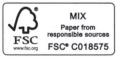

MIX
Paper from
responsible sources
FSC® C018575
www.fsc.org

Library of Congress Control Number: 2012939478

British Library Cataloguing in Publication data

A catalogue record for this book is available from
the British Library

ISBN 978-0-85702-547-0
ISBN 978-0-85702-548-7 (pbk)

Contents

About the Authors

Joanna De Souza MSc BSc RGN PATHE

Joanna De Souza has a professional background as a Clinical Nurse Specialist with specific expertise in bone marrow transplantation and end-of-life care. She is currently a Lecturer at Kings College London where she teaches on cancer and end-of-life care issues across the education provision from the pre-registration to Master's level programs. Joanna is particularly interested in the development of creative learning modalities and in supporting wider access students.

Her clinical practice links, teaching and research interests are in the field of end-of-life care and have involved working in a variety of care settings in both UK and South Island, New Zealand.

Annie Pettifer MSc, BSc, PGCEA, RGN

Annie Pettifer has worked extensively as a Clinical Nurse Specialist in end-of-life care across both the acute and community settings. She has also worked as a District Nurse. She is currently a Senior Lecturer in Adult Nursing at Coventry University where she teaches end-of-life care education across pre-registration and continuing professional development.

She is particularly interested in the teaching of communication skills and spirituality in pre-registration nurses and has recently developed bespoke education in end-of-life care for ambulance clinicians.

Acknowledgements

We would like to thank our friends and family with particular thanks to Adam and Roger for their support and tolerance of our long hours in front of a computer. Thanks also to our parents: John and Valerie Pettifer for their outstanding proof-reading and meticulous attention to the peculiarities of the English language and to Joy and Harold De Souza for their ambitious inspiration and enthusiasm. We thank everyone at Sage for ongoing patience and support on the steep learning curve of writing for book publication. We could not have completed this task without a multitude of people at Kings College, London and Coventry University who started us on this journey, offered support, survival skills, time and the incentive to complete the work. Our thanks go to the many patients and families we have nursed. They taught immeasurably by sharing their experiences of dying and it is this knowledge which we now share through this book. Finally we would like to thank the inspirational nurse lecturers of South Bank Polytechnic who taught us as student nurses. We hope this book, by the pair at the front who asked endless questions, would make them smile!

Introduction

Caring for people approaching the end of their lives can be daunting for students, particularly those meeting this situation for the first time (Higginson 2006; Parry 2011). Students care deeply that the end-of-life care they offer is of a high quality but lack confidence in how to achieve this. Students' concerns are likely to include being anxious about what to say to patients and relatives, and how they might cope with witnessing death, perhaps for the first time.

A desire to offer good quality care is important but it is not sufficient in itself. Patients and relatives need nurses who have the skill and knowledge to ease the difficulties that end of life can bring. Therefore, nurses and all health and social care professionals need evidence-based knowledge to apply to the situations they encounter in practice. This book focuses on equipping students with the knowledge they need to care confidently for patients approaching the end of their lives.

The approach of the book

This book uses case studies to illustrate challenges that occur in practice. Whilst each case is unique, the case studies as a whole reflect key issues that may arise in this area of practice. The book pinpoints pertinent research and theory, and, drawing on the authors' own experience as palliative care specialists and educators, analyses the issues in depth. The knowledge gained through such exploration is applied to each case as a practical example of end-of-life care. The appropriate role and expectations of nurses in each case is teased out and emphasised, thus equipping students with both underpinning knowledge and practical strategies to confidently deliver end-of-life care.

The structure of the book

Chapter 1 End-of-life care – a historical perspective offers a short historical account of the development of palliative and end-of-life care including the development of the National End-of-Life Care Strategy. This is illustrated through a historical case study of woman, Bridget, who is dying in her home in 1880. By tracing the context in which end-of-life care was delivered at that time, the chapter explores the changes in the delivery of end-of-life care and how there are plans to improve the quality end-of-life care for all in the future.

Chapter 2 Assessing holistic needs considers the vital area of assessment in depth including what should be assessed and how this might be achieved. It draws on the case of Mr Clarkson, a man with complex needs at the end of life for whom a holistic assessment has been requested.

Chapter 3 Responding to questions about the end of life focuses on communication. Strategies and approaches that enable or hinder communication are explored through practical examples. The chapter also discusses how bad news might be broken sensitively. The topic is explored through the case of Mary, who asks the student caring for her in hospital difficult questions about the end of her life.

Chapter 4 Making difficult choices using ethical and legal frameworks presents the dilemma of whether or not treatment is appropriate in the case of Edith, an older woman with multi-infarct dementia living in a nursing home. Key ethical principles are applied to Edith's case and pertinent legal guidance is explained. The role of the student in such difficult decision-making is made clear.

Chapter 5 Calling in the palliative care team explores the different types of palliative care approaches and considers when it may be appropriate to refer to specialist palliative care through the case of Bert, an older man with chronic renal failure. It explores some of the different roles that professionals in the multi-diciplinary team may play in the delivery of end-of-life care.

Chapter 6 Managing physical symptoms considers some of the common symptoms experienced by patients approaching the end of life through the case of Aarti Shah who has advanced breast cancer. The chapter explores essential principles of symptom management.

Chapter 7 Discharging patients approaching the end of life details the discharge of Mr Sevim from hospital to home in line with his wishes. It equips the reader with practical knowledge of how to plan the discharge of someone who wishes to go home to die.

Chapter 8 Knowing when a patient is in the last days of life explores the difficult issues of identifying whe someone is dying and then the management of some of symptoms patients may experience at this time of life through the case study of Reg, an older man with congestive cardiac failure. The chapter explores the development of end-of-life care pathways.

Chapter 9 Care after death looks at the care of patients and their families at the point of death and in the first few days after death by considering the case of Mrs Dorothy Graham who dies at home and the experience of her husband Bill. This includes some exploration of what this experience may feel like for someone who has not been with someone at the time at which they die.

Chapter 10 Sudden or unexpected death focuses on the added complexity when death is unexpected with a focus on the sudden death of Bupa on an intensive care unit and the care of his family. It explores issues such as the challenges we may face in notifying families of the death and how sudden death may complicate bereavement for those involved.

Chapter 11 Supporting family and friends considers the effect of loss and bereavement for our patients and their families at the end of life and outlines some of the models of loss that have helped to shape our understanding of the experiences of families and friends. The chapter looks at the case study of a dying widow, Lydia, and her children offers suggestions for how we can offer sensitive and appropriate support.

Chapter 12 Resolving my own feelings after a patient has died focuses on the impact that end-of-life care may have on students and healthcare professionals. The case study describes the impact of Mark's sudden death on Peter, a student nurse. Understanding what commonly motivates professionals to care, and the impact caring might have on them, may help students to develop personal resilience to the sadness associated with end-of-life care whilst remaining compassionate. Helpful strategies that promote the well-being of students are discussed.

Professional regulation context

This book is underpinned by each of the seven steps within the End-of-Life Care Pathway (Department of Health 2008) below:

- Step 1:   Identifying people approaching the end of life.
- Step 2:   Care planning: assessing needs and preferences, agreeing a care plan to reflect these and reviewing these regularly.
- Step 3:   Co-ordination of care.
- Step 4:   Delivery of high quality services in all locations.
- Step 5:   Management of the last days of life.
- Step 6:   Care after death.
- Step 7:   Support for carers, both during a person's illness and after their death.

Chapter 1 includes some discussion around **Step 1: Identifying people approaching the end of life.** The End-of-Life Care Strategy (Department of Health 2008) called for a concerted approach amongst all health care staff in recognising when someone may be approaching the end of their life and initiating appropriate discussion about this with them. Chapters 3 and 4 look at how some of the difficult conversations around end of life may be handled and the ethical decisions that may need to be made through these conversations.

Chapter 2 explores assessment in end of life care and addresses **Step 2: Care planning** including how to take into consideration patients' own preferences about the care they would like to receive. Chapter 7 looks at the need to plan efficiently to enable these preferences to be achieved, particularly when circumstances may be changing quickly. Chapter 6 goes on to look at how care can be planned around patient choices and care needs.

Chapter 5 focuses on **Step 3: Co-ordination of care.** It is important that people receive the most appropriate care for their needs and that those caring for them are aware of how and when to appropriately access specialist palliative care.

With regards to **Step 4: Delivery of high quality services in all locations,** the book is designed to offer perspectives from several different care settings. Chapter 7 deals in particular with the issues of changing settings, using a scenario of someone being discharged from hospital into the community.

Chapter 8 explores **Step 5: Management of the last days of life.** This includes discussion of some of the tools available to help provide good care at this point such as the end-of-life care pathways.

Chapter 9 considers **Step 6: Care after death** and the issues that arise when this is complicated by sudden or unexpected death are addressed Chapter 10.

Step 7: Support for carers, both during a person's illness and after their death is covered in Chapter 10 by looking at the reactions to loss from by family and carers during a person's final illness and through their death. Chapter 12 addresses the needs of professional carers working with people facing these multiple losses as part of their daily role.

In addition, the book addresses the Nursing and Midwifery Council (NMC) Generic Standards for Competence (NMC 2010) as shown below:

1 Professional values.
2 Communication and interpersonal skills.
3 Nursing practice and decision-making.
4 Leadership management and team working.

1. Professional values

The importance of maintaining people's dignity by respecting their autonomy and right to self-determination is an underpinning value throughout the book and features in each chapter, with emphasis placed on empowering people to be more actively involved in the decisions being made about the options available to them. In particular, Chapters 2 and 4 explore how we might do this with consideration of understanding the ethical principles involved.

2. Communication and interpersonal skills

The theme of communication again threads through the book, starting with effective assessment in Chapter 2 and dealing with challenging conversations in Chapter 3.

3. Nursing practice and decision-making

The assessment, planning and evaluation of care are core features of the book. All the chapters take a patient scenario and consider through the chapter how care needs may be elicited and assessed, care may be planned and in many cases elements of how it may be evaluated.

4. Leadership management and team working

Encouraging student nurses to be involved in helping with care decisions and playing an active part in the health care team are core parts of Chapters 4, 6, 7 and 8. Having a greater understanding of their own needs and those of carers and family members in Chapters 10 and 11 equips student nurses to develop good management and leadership skills as they move towards registration and full staff nurse responsibilities.

Learning features

Each chapter poses Reflective Questions for the reader to consider their own experience and their future approach to end-of-life care, based on the knowledge they have learned from the chapter. Action Points are also provided to encourage readers to apply the evidence to practice situations. These features can be considered by individuals working alone or within groups that may be facilitated by a teacher.

Moreover, the chapters direct readers to literature, useful research websites and sources within the arts, literature and films which to assist students in expanding their knowledge further.

Looking to the future

Whilst caring for patients approaching the end of their lives is undoubtedly challenging, the development of end of life care skills for nurses and healthcare professionals offers a real hope that patients and their families will be cared for to a high standard. For students themselves, caring for patients approaching the end of their life offers the privilege of sharing significantly in the lives of many patients and families at a time of great loss and change. It can be a poignant reminder of the value of the life ahead of the living, challenging all to live it to the full.

References

Department of Health (2008) *End-of-Life Care Strategy: Promoting High Quality Care for All Adults at the End of Life.* London: Deparment of Health.

Higginson, R. (2006) 'Fears, worries and experiences of first year pre-registration nursing students: a qualitative study', *Nurse Research* 13 (3): 32–49.

Nursing and Midwifery Council (2010) *Standards for Pre-Registration Nursing Education.* London: Nursing and Midwifery Council.

Parry, M. (2011) 'Student nurses' experience of their first death in clinical practice International', *Journal of Palliative Nursing,* 17 (9): 448–453.

CHAPTER 1

End-of-life care – a historical perspective

Joanna De Souza with Annie Pettifer

This chapter will explore:

- How professional care of the dying has developed over the last century
- The philosophy of palliative care
- What we mean by the term 'end of life'
- The End of Life Care Strategy
- How it might be different to be dying today

Introduction

The places where people die have changed markedly over the past century with most deaths no longer occurring at home but in hospital. In around 1900 about 85% of people died in their own homes, with workhouses accounting for most other deaths. By the mid-twentieth century around 50% of people died at home. In the early twenty-first century acute hospitals have become the most common place of death. (Department of Health 2008a)

Our first chapter will discuss the concept of end of life and explore the context of caring for those at the end of their lives and the influences that shape the care that is offered.

We will start from a historical perspective with a case presentation from the past, and trace how care of the dying has developed over the last century in response to changes in health care and society as a whole. As the story becomes current we will consider how end of life and end-of-life care is now defined. We will consider how government policy shapes the care in differing organisations and current initiatives which seek to develop end-of-life care provision.

Bridget

Bridget is a 39 year-old married woman living with her husband and five surviving children aged between 18 months and 17 years. She lives in a small cottage in a rural village north of Leeds where she and her family are agricultural labourers on the estate farm. The year is 1880.

Bridget has had a troublesome cough for a short while now and expectorates sputum with traces of blood in it. Over the last couple of days she has become weak and has been unable to get out of bed. She has a fever with night sweats, flushed cheeks and bright eyes. She cannot eat.

Her family have seen this many times before. They know she has consumption and that she may die soon, as have many others in the village. They close the shutters of the cottage, light candles and call the vicar. Many family members, neighbours and friends call in so that the cottage is often full.

Bridget's last days and nights are beset with coughing and a growing breathlessness as she loses the strength to cough any more.

Bridget's family lay out the body after she has died and she remains in the house until the next day when a funeral is held. She is placed in a rough wooden coffin and this is carried down the street by the men of the family to the church. Being a regular churchgoer, she is buried in a shared grave at the back of the church graveyard. Most of the village turn out to pay their respects as Bridget's family are well known.

How professional care of the dying has developed over the last century

The case study above typifies common death in nineteenth-century Britain. In 1891–1900 life expectancy was 44 years for men and 47 years for women and in 1880 33% of those deaths were due to infectious and parasitic diseases. Indeed some 80,000 people died of consumption (now called Tuberculosis or TB) (Office for National Statistics 1998; House of Commons, 1999). Like Bridget, most people died at home after a short illness, cared for by family, neighbours and friends who would have been familiar with the process of dying. Professional health care would have been unavailable to the vast majority. The only professionals who would have played a significant role would have been the clergy.

Dedicated institutionalised care for the dying, in the form of hospices, dates back to 1842. Previous to this, and over the centuries, there had been places that offered care to the poor, ill and destitute, but many died without any kind of professional support. The idea of a specific place focusing on those in the last weeks of life was not well known. The word 'hospice' was first applied to the care of dying patients by a widow, Mme Garnier, who founded the Dames de Calaire in France, in 1842. Other hospices followed, including one established for the poor in Nottingham in 1877 by Mary Potter, a Catholic nun. It was served by the first Catholic order of nuns in the UK, her Little Company of Mary. Mary Potter herself suffered from what was thought to be a terminal episode of illness, but she recovered and was inspired to provide some solace for others (Tothill, 1999). Nuns continued to be the major providers of end-of-life care with the opening of hospices such as Trinity Hospice (originally the Hostel of God) in 1891 and St Joseph's hospice in London in 1905.

Reflective questions

What might it have been like to care for someone like Bridget and her family, where there would have been no running water and very little access to any equipment or medications?

Palliative care in some parts of the world still reflects this reality. How much do we take the environment and tools we have for granted?

As the twentieth century progressed, the manner in which people died and the way dying people were cared for changed, reflecting shifts in society as the world became more industrialised and people moved to urban living. With the establishment of the National Health Service in 1948, professional health care was now available to all. By 1957, 45% of deaths occurred in hospitals (Ariès 1991) and with this came a diminishment in familiarity with death and caring for the dying previously held within the community. Many widespread infectious diseases, such as consumption, which our patient Bridget suffered from, were now treatable and people were dying from more protracted illness such as cancer. This meant that they needed more care for a longer period before death.

In the first 20 years after the creation of the NHS the experience of the dying was explored by a number of physicians seeking to improve the care offered to those close to death. John Hinton (1963), who went on to be an influential part of the modern hospice movement, documents that Osler, known by some as the father of modern medicine, as early as 1906, studied the symptoms of the dying. Hinton conducted his own studies in the early 1960s (Hinton 1963). He suggested that perhaps there had been little previous identification of the needs of the dying due to the difficulties of having conversations about dying between physicians and patients. He noted that in his study, which allowed patients to drive the conversation about what troubled them most, patients were so often relieved to be allowed to talk about their feelings and personal problems.

Hinton's findings included the high prevalence of depression, physical and other mental distress, and also a need for care which included holistic elements such as spirituality. He also found that the majority of patients who were considered to be eligible to be referred to his end-of-life study had cancer. In his paper in 1963, he surmised that others were not referred partly due to the difficulty in diagnosing the dying phase of other illnesses, but also because their care was always more treatment orientated. His findings are hauntingly reflective of modern studies looking at the needs of dying patients, now more than 40 years later.

However, it may be argued that the course of modern end-of-life care was perhaps most heavily influenced by a young girl born in London in 1918. Cicely Saunders (later to become Dame Cicely Saunders), following a difficult school life, entered Cambridge to study Politics, Philosophy and Economics just before the Second World War. However, wanting to assist in the relief of the suffering she saw around her, she left her course to train as a Red Cross nurse at the Nightingale School of Nursing. A back injury led her out of nursing and to train as a medical almoner (a kind of social worker). She went on to work in London, where she used her new role to work with people with cancer in St Luke's hospital (Du Boulay 2007). She found herself challenged by the patients she cared for, and in particular by a Polish patient – David Tasma – who she came to love and with whom she worked up to his death. She discussed with him her dreams of improving the care of dying patients by seeking to look after not only their physical needs but also their psychological and spiritual needs. David Tasma left her £500 to start a home for dying patients. Motivated by this, she embarked on medical training, qualifying as a medical doctor in 1957, and then used her training to enter the world of pharmacology and research.

Dame Cicely's research interests were naturally in the control of pain in the terminally ill. While working at St Mary's Hospital in London as a researcher, she explored the link between dependency on morphine and its administration, and demonstrated that regular low doses of morphine alleviated patients' pain more effectively than the fewer, higher doses which had hitherto been administered to the dying. This research contributed to the World Health Organisation pain philosophy and changed the experience of the dying forever (WHO 2006).

Dame Cicely then began a period of 10 years of research into the care of the dying at St Joseph's Hospice in Hackney – one of the very few homes for dying people at that time. Many of the common practices in care of the dying that we see today result from the work she undertook there, including the introduction of the total pain model which highlighted the need to look holistically when considering pain relief at the end of life.

In addition to her clinical and research roles, Dame Cicely, inspired and supported by two more Polish men, one of whom she eventually married, worked at raising awareness and funding to open the St Christopher's Hospice in South London in 1967. Initially an inpatient facility, home visits and day care services and were quickly established, and St Christopher's Hospice became the prototype model for modern hospices and palliative care in the UK and internationally. Through extensive outreach, research and educational endeavour, care of the dying became a growing health care speciality. Cicely Saunders was made a Dame Commander of the British Empire in 1980 and was awarded Britain's Order of Merit in 1989 for her services to health care.

The philosophy of palliative care

The word 'palliative' is derived from the Latin word 'paliere', which means to cloak or shield. It may be considered, therefore, as an approach to care which aims to mitigate or shield someone from the distressing effects a serious illness has on them. *The Oxford Dictionary* (2012) defines 'palliation' more simply as:

> intent to alleviate a problem without addressing the underlying cause.

In essence, then, palliative care is simply an approach to caring for someone which aims to alleviate the effects of a disease rather than disease itself. It is summed up by the most widely used definition, by the World Health Organisation, first in 1989 and through several revisions to this current definition:

> Palliative care is an approach that improves the quality of life of patients and their families facing the problems associated with life-threatening illness, through the prevention and relief of suffering by means of early identification and impeccable assessment and treatment of pain and other problems, physical, psychosocial and spiritual. (WHO 2012)

Such definitions clearly show that palliative care may be helpful to all those with advanced progressive illness regardless of their diagnosis, age or circumstances.

The impetus started by Dame Cicely led to the development of a whole movement in palliative care. Initially, nurses were more receptive to her holistic philosophy than the medical profession (Clark 2008) and in the first couple of decades the modern palliative care movement was nurse-led. In the UK, palliative care also developed as a speciality that crossed the traditionally fixed institutional contexts. Palliative care teams worked in hospitals, hospices and in the community, often with strong links between them as they were based next to each other to facilitate better communication. Voluntary sector organisations – in particular Macmillan and Marie Curie Cancer Care – also played a major role in how palliative care developed, while other organisations, such as Help the Hospices and the National Council for Palliative Care, became major players particularly focusing on issues of funding and policy. Doctors then increasingly became more involved and more influential in the decision-making processes, and in the late 1980s palliative care was officially recognised as a medical speciality. However, it has remained a speciality that is recognisable by its strong tradition of multidisciplinary working and leadership.

The effect of AIDS on the development of palliative care

Although palliative care developed as a speciality focusing mainly on cancer in the UK, in the early 1980s a new disease – human immunodeficiency virus (HIV), known then as AIDS (acquired immunodeficiency syndrome) – emerged that diversified its focus. It was first recognised as a major end-of-life illness in the USA but soon became a disease affecting much of the western world.

In 1988, the Mildmay Mission in London, which had previously been more of a mission hospital, became Europe's first dedicated AIDS hospice. This was closely followed by the London Lighthouse. While it is not easy to trace some of the detail about this type of palliative care, as these documents are now harder to access, Armes and Higginson (1999) illustrate how this group of patients and their carers were looking for a type of palliative care that sat much more comfortably alongside more acute treatment modalities, such as artificial feeding and hydration, and active medical treatments than perhaps had been the case up until that time.

As knowledge and treatments for HIV infection have evolved, it has become much less of an end-of-life diagnosis in the western/developed world. However, it has become a major concern and driver for the development of palliative care in the developing world where, due to a lack of financial resources, education, treatment and palliation of people with HIV infection has been much more complicated and insufficient. As a result the disease has spread, creating a huge need for HIV palliative care services across the world.

Reflective question

As a nurse working in the last century, if you were not working in oncology or HIV you would have limited access to the services of a palliative care team. There were no tools available such as the end-of-life care pathways and the support of organisations such as hospices. Macmillan and Marie Curie were not available outside these specialities. How do you think this might have affected the care you would have been able to give dying patients you were caring for in other areas?

Palliative care in the new millennium

In the UK, Calman and Hine (Expert Advisory Group on Cancer 1995), in their report on cancer services, called for a more integrated approach and for palliative care to be seen much more as a supportive therapy along the course of a disease trajectory, rather than simply care around the time of dying.

As health care provision in the UK prepared to enter the new millennium, global collaboration had taken off with the development of the internet and online communication. This resulted in new treatments for many diseases and a growth in the culture of the need to cure.

In 2003 only 8.5% of those dying from cancer over age 85 died in hospice compared with 20% for all ages (Seymour et al. 2005). Other inequities were also found to exist. In 2006 only 7.2% of patients in specialist services had a non-malignant diagnosis (National Council for Palliative Care 2006). Inequalities around disenfranchised groups within the cancer population were also a concern, such as the work highlighting the lack of access by black and ethnic minority groups (BME) (Koffman and Higginson 2001). A review of the palliative care literature between 1995 and 2005 indicated a widespread concern about these inequities, with a very uneven emphasis being placed on offering services to those dying of cancer. There was a mounting need to address these issues in a national way and this led to the development of a number of palliative care tools which were to change the provision of palliative care, particularly in the UK, quite dramatically. These included the Liverpool Care Pathway, the Gold Standards Framework and the Marie Curie Preferred Place of Care tool. All of these tools are discussed in further detail in later chapters in the book.

There were a number of different reasons for this unequal distribution. In the UK, one major aspect was the funding sources of palliative care provision (Dunlop 2001). Much of the funding for the provision of palliative care came from voluntary giving by both organisations and individuals. This type of funding tends to be different in different parts of the country and what it is spent on is often chosen by those who are donating. This may account for why much of the provision remained cancer-focused. Cancer is a disease that creates a great deal of anxiety as it is seen as a disease that can affect anyone, unexpectedly and often having a profound effect on their lives. As a result it attracts a large amount of voluntary donations. Other diseases lack some of the anxiety and notoriety attributed to cancer so attract fewer donations.

However, a growing voice of concern about the lack of ability to provide good care even to those with a cancer diagnosis at the end of life was highlighted in the Cancer Plan from the Department of Health (2000a). The Plan called for a much greater commitment of government funding to ensure more universal provision of palliative care. In 2003 the government committed to £50 million per year of funding into improving palliative and end-of-life care. Although primarily this was for funding into improving palliative care in cancer, the funding was also available to bids seeking to improve the care of people requiring palliative care for other conditions.

Internationally, palliative care also saw a real growth around the millennium. Events such as the opening up of the Iron Curtain and Eastern Europe saw a new need for palliative care, particularly in the care of children with disabilities. It was estimated that around 100 million people worldwide were in need of palliative care (Stjernsward and Clark 2004). Services were being developed, particularly in English-speaking areas, but provision worldwide was patchy (Wright 2004).

Moving forward

In light of the growing evidence of a need for change, the National End of Life Care Programme was set up in 2004. It incorporated the newly developed end-of-life care tools, a drive for increasing end-of-life care education among all health care providers regardless of speciality, and a desire to widen the scope of end-of-life care provision from its cancer base. One of the features of this programme was to redefine what end-of-life care was. We see here the terminology start to change from palliative care to end-of-life care (McGinn 2010).

What we mean by the term 'End of Life'

Reflection questions

When do you think someone is at the end of life?

Is it in those last few days before they die and perhaps are placed on the end-of-life care pathway?

Think of some of the elderly patients you have cared for. How long would you have considered them to have been at the end of their lives? Is it different for different patients? What sort of factors make you feel differently about different patients?

Human development in psychosocial terms is a continuous process from birth through to preparation for death. Erik Erikson (1998), a psychoanalyst, proposed a series of eight developmental stages that people go through as they progressed through life. Erikson proposes that the last and eighth psychosocial stage, ego integrity versus despair, begins when a person has a sense that they are entering their last stage of life and are approaching death. This awareness of impending death precipitates the final life crisis. This last life crisis involves conducting a review of their lives and determining if it was a success or failure. That is, ego integrity occurs if one can have a sense of satisfaction or can come to terms with how they have lived so far. He suggests that this tends to happen in older age but may also be linked with significant life events, such as retirement, the death of a spouse or close friends, or the diagnosis of a life-limiting illness.

Having an awareness that one is reaching the end of life allows one to start to engage with this process of life review and also perhaps some of the adjustments that one may want to make to relationships, property arrangements and just things one may want to accomplish before one dies. The film, *The Bucket List* (2007), tells the story of a man who had a list of things he wanted to achieve before he died and the film is a humorous account of how, when faced with death, he sought to achieve some of these and, perhaps most importantly, was able to work through some of the unresolved relationship difficulties he had had with significant people in his life.

Dr Keri Thomas, who developed the Gold Standards Framework (GSF), urged a wider sense of thinking around the time when one might be considered end of life. She suggested that perhaps this may involve months or even years in a person with an advanced irreversible illness, rather than just the last few weeks (McGinn 2010). Her programme involves encouraging general practitioners and community teams to be identifying patients who are in this last stage of life (i.e. those who may be in the last year of life), and using the monthly GSF meetings to consider their health needs in a proactive way to try to promote more choice at the end of life and to prevent unnecessary admissions to hospital. This is discussed in further detail in Chapter 7.

The role of hope in end-of-life care

Clayton et al. (2008) conducted a systematic review into sustaining hope when working with terminally ill patients. They found evidence that many patients seem to be able to maintain a sense of hope despite acknowledging the terminal nature of their illness. Both patients and relatives valued honesty from professionals and that professionals may help patients to cope with impending death by exploring and fostering realistic forms of hope that are meaningful for the particular patient and their family. Calman (1984), a very experienced oncologist, proposed a model which has become known as the Calman Gap. If we can narrow the gap between expectation and reality for patients and relatives it will result in increased quality of life (Figure 1.1).

Since its proposal a number of studies have been undertaken to explore this hypothesis. What has been revealed is that there is some validity to this concept although it is helpful to have hope to tolerate difficult treatments (Higginson 2000). There are also cultural questions that still need to be explored about the contradiction that occurs between clarifying expectations and religious and cultural patterns of non-disclosure of life-threatening diagnoses that exists in some communities.

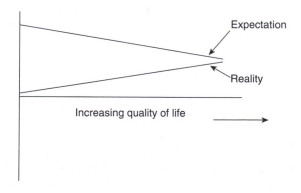

Figure 1.1   The Calman Gap

Initiating discussions – does it remove hope?

Initiating discussions about the fact that a patient may be dying is nearly always difficult. Some of the concerns held by professionals in this area are discussed more fully in Chapters 2 and 3. However, concerns about taking away people's hope often result in these conversations not being initiated by professionals until patients are reaching very late stages of their disease. Clayton et al.'s (2008) review of sustaining hope at the end of life offers an alternative perspective. Jenko et al. (2007) discuss how more open disclosure and the process of initiating discussions early enough can allow for a period of time during which people can do some form of life review, making sense of their life even when it is coming to a close prematurely. Following in the ideology of Erikson and Erikson (1998), this may allow them to have conversations, have significant times with loved ones or put right situations from their pasts. Trueman and Parker (2006) offer an interesting study on how community nurses can engage in facilitative life review with the patients they are caring for who are coming to the end of their lives. Perhaps this process can also contribute to revising life goals and facilitating hope at the end of life.

Reflective questions

Having read the discussions so far, consider what you now understand by the terms 'end of life' or 'palliative care'. You might like to make a note of your thoughts and refer to them as you progress through this book.

Think about some of the hopes your patients may have that may be achievable even when at the end of life? How might you explore these with them?

The End of Life Care Strategy

For some years in the UK there had been a call for a government strategy that focused solely on palliative and end-of-life care. Palliative care had been a part of many documents, such as the Cancer Plan (Department of Health 2000a) and the NICE guidelines for supportive care in cancer (2004), and as an element of several of the National Service Frameworks, such as the NSF on chronic heart disease and long-term conditions (Department of Health, 2000b; 2005) The importance of end-of-life care in the Labour government's health strategy was highlighted in the publication of Lord Darzi's report, *The Next Stage Review* (Department of Health, 2007). This report was produced for the government to evaluate the impact of the NHS plan and labour policy 10 years after they were elected in 1997. The report cited 'End of Life Care' as one of the eight clinical pathways developed by each of the Strategic Health Authorities in England. Finally, in 2008 the Department of Health produced a long-awaited End of Life Care Strategy (Department of Health 2008a).

The aim of the strategy is to provide people approaching the end of life with more choice about where they would like to live and die. It is designed to encompass all adults with advanced, progressive illness and care given in all settings (Department of Health 2008a).

An important aspect of modern palliative care, through the setting of national (where possible) standards and guidelines is that the best care is available to all who require it regardless of where in the country they live. In the report (Department of Health 2008a), Travers and Mitchell explain how the UK Departments of England, Scotland and Wales have chosen to do this in different ways. Scotland has opted for mandatory clinical standards whereas England and Wales have chosen guidelines developed through NICE. The End of Life Care impact assessment document (Department of Health 2008b) specifies the areas and types of assessment that are required to make progress with this.

The themes covered in the strategy were informed by over 300 other stakeholders (people and organisations who have an interest in palliative care), including all the major palliative care organisations both in the NHS and the voluntary sector. A clear care pathway was produced for both the commissioning (planning and paying for) and the delivery of care. This care pathway consisted of seven steps:

- Identification of people approaching the end of life and initiating discussions about preferences for end-of-life care;
- Care planning: assessing needs and preferences, agreeing a care plan to reflect these and reviewing these regularly;
- Co-ordination of care;
- Delivery of high-quality services in all locations;
- Management of the last days of life;
- Care after death; and
- Support for carers, both during a person's illness and after their death.

How can we use the strategy to improve the care that we give? The strategy highlights key areas that need to be addressed in the provision of end-of-life care across the country and offers recommendations about how this may be done. Some of the areas which are highlighted in the strategy are discussed below.

The strategy encourages raising the profile of end-of-life care and is aimed at getting people to talk about dying. It is hoped that it will make it less of a taboo subject in society. This will hopefully pave the way to enabling more discussion and awareness of the choices people have about where and how they die. The National Council for Palliative Care has played a large role with the general public in this respect, with their campaign *Dying Matters* (NCPC 2012).

One of the first priorities of the strategy is for a concerted approach of education and awareness-raising of all health care staff who may care for someone at the end of life to recognise when someone may be entering this phase of life and to initiating some appropriate discussions with them. To help people decide when this might be, the strategy introduces 'the surprise question'. If you can answer 'no' to this question about a patient, then it is time to start having end-of-life conversations:

Would you be surprised if this person was to die in the next year?

Too often these conversations have been started too late or only started after the patient has raised the issues. Chapters 2 and 3 explore issues around communication at the end of life and some of these perhaps difficult conversations.

Other priorities highlighted by the strategy are the issues around assessment and planning of end-of-life care. It explores who should be giving care, including decisions about when to refer patients to specialist palliative care teams and how to ensure good communication between all professionals involved in delivering the care. This needs to extend across the boundaries of hospital, community teams and those working in care homes so as more people express a wish about where they would like to die, health and social care services need to be able to respond quickly and communication channels need to be clearly established to facilitate situations such as people leaving hospital to die at home. They encourage the use of end-of-life tools to facilitate good deaths for as many people as possible, many of which will be discussed through the course of this book.

The strategy highlights the importance of the role of family and informal carers during this phase of life. It calls for the provision of care for these people to be a key part of the end-of-life care pathway. The needs of family and informal carers facing loss are explored in Chapter 11. However, it is also important to consider the needs of the health care professionals, as formal carers, and this issue is addressed in Chapter 12.

The strategy recognises that the education of all staff involved is imperative if the aims of this strategy are to be achieved. It develops the terminology from specialist and generalist providers, coined by the NICE guidelines in supportive care (2004), to dividing staff into three groups: (1) staff who spend the whole of their time caring for those at the end of life; (2) staff who frequently deal with end-of-life care as part of their role; and (3) staff who care for people at the end of life infrequently, recognising that the educational needs and core competencies required of these staff will differ.

How it might be different to be dying today

Returning to our case study at the beginning of this chapter, if Bridget was dying in the UK today, she would probably have been dying of something very different. It is very unusual for people of Bridget's age to die at all in the UK. However, at her age breast cancer is the most common cause of death. It is likely that Bridget would be at the end of a number of treatments for her cancer, having had a mix of inpatient and outpatient chemotherapy, radiotherapy and hormone therapy.

Bridget would hopefully have a range of choices about where she wanted to die, including at the hospital in which she was treated, at home under the care of district and community palliative care nurses, in a local hospice offering a wide range of supportive care, or in a place that was special to her for some other reason. In the UK, it is the aim of the health services to be able to provide Bridget with the palliative and end-of-life care, free at the point of need, wherever she may choose to die.

We hope this book will help to equip you on your journey to being able to offer high-quality, personalised and compassionate end-of-life care in partnership with this technologically developing world.

Summary

In summary, the key points to remember when considering the origins and current direction of palliative and end-of-life care are:

- The manner in which people die, has changed over the past 100 years. Since the 1960s, through Cicely Saunders' extraordinary story, we have seen the development of the modern hospice movement and a growth in the training and provision of specialist care in all settings where people are being cared for at the end of life.
- One of the challenges of providing good end-of-life care has been a need to ensure better awareness of who is at the end of life and the needs that they may have.
- A second challenge is to ensure that palliative care services are responsive to the needs of all who are dying and not just those dying of certain diseases.
- The last decade has seen the development of a National End of Life Care Programme which incorporates a number of tools to help ensure better delivery of end-of-life care. As a result of these, together with the work of many, we now have an End of Life Care Strategy for the UK.
- Knowing how to access and to understand the scope of what services are available will enable us to provide a high level of end-of-life care.

Further reading

As you start your journey into the exploration of developing the care you can offer to patients who are coming to the end of their lives and their families, it will be useful to familiarise yourself with the National End of Life Care Programme and, in particular, the pages looking at the End of Life Care Strategy. These can be found at www.endoflifecareforadults.nhs.uk/strategy.

For a more detailed exploration of the historical origins of palliative care, you may want to read David Clark's historical article in *The Lancet Oncology* (Clark 2007). Reading Salimah Meghani's (2003) paper looking at the development of palliative care in the USA offers an interesting contrast.

Several films look at the issues of people approaching the end of life, such as: *Life as a House* (2001), with Hayden Christensen, Kevin Kline and Kristin Scott Thomas, and *The Bucket List* (2007), with Jack Nicholson and Morgan Freeman, which are both about coming to the end of life with unfinished business to complete. *Philadelphia* (1993), starring Tom

Hanks and Denzel Washington, offers an insight into the early days of the AIDS epidemic of the 1980s and the effect it had on those who were diagnosed with the syndrome.

References

Ariès, P. (1991) *The Hour of Our Death*. Oxford: Oxford University Press.

Armes, P.J. and Higginson, I.J. (1999) 'What constitutes high-quality HIV/AIDS palliative care?', *Journal Palliative Care*, 15(4): 5–12.

Calman, K. (1984) 'Quality of life in cancer patients: an hypothesis', *Journal of Medical Ethics*, 10: 124–7.

Clark, D. (2007) 'From margins to centre: a review of the history of palliative care in cancer', *The Lancet Oncology*, 8(5): 430–8.

Clark, D. (2008) 'History and culture in the rise of palliative care', Chapter 2 in S. Payne, J. Seymour and C. Ingleton (eds), *Palliative Care Nursing: Principles and Evidence for Practice* (2nd edn). Milton Keynes: Open University Press.

Clayton, J.M., Hancock, K., Parker, S., Butow, P.N., Walder, S., Carrick, S., Currow, D., Ghersi, D., Glare, P., Hagerty, R., Olver, I.N. and Tattersall, M.H. (2008) 'Sustaining hope when communicating with terminally ill patients and their families: a systematic review', *Psychooncology*, 17(7): 641–59.

Department of Health (2000a) *The NHS Cancer Plan: A Plan for Investment, a Plan for Reform*. London: Department of Health.

Department of Health (2000b) *National Service Framework for Coronary Heart Disease*. London: Department of Health.

Department of Health (2005) *National Service Framework for Long Term Conditions*. London: Department of Health.

Department of Health (2007) *Our NHS, Our Future: NHS Next Stage Review – Interim Report*. London: Department of Health.

Department of Health (2008a) *End of Life Care Strategy: Promoting High Quality Care for All Adults at the End of Life*. London: Department of Health.

Department of Health (2008b) *End of Life Care Strategy: Promoting High Quality Care for All Adults at the End of Life, Equality Impact Assessment*. London: Department of Health.

Du Boulay, S. (2007) *Cicely Saunders: The Founder of the Modern Hospice Movement*. London: SPCK Publishing.

Dunlop, R. (2001) 'Specialist palliative care and non-malignant diseases', Chapter 2 in J.M. Addington-Hall and I.J. Higginson (eds), *Palliative Care for Non-Cancer Patients*. Oxford: Oxford University Press.

Erikson, E. and Erikson, J. (1998) *The Life Cycle Completed*. New York: W.W. Norton & Company.

Expert Advisory Group on Cancer (1995) *A Policy Framework for Commissioning Cancer Services* (Calman–Hine Report). London: Department of Health.

Higginson, I. (2000) 'The quality of expectation: healing palliation or disappointment', *Journal of the Royal Society of Medicine*, 93(12): 609–10.

Hinton, J. (1963) 'The physical and mental distress of the dying', *Quarterly Journal of Medicine*, 32: 1–21.

House of Commons (1999) *A Century of Change: Trends in UK Statistics since 1900*. Research paper 99/111. London: House of Commons.

Jenko, M., Gonzalez, L. and Seymour, M. (2007) 'Life review with the terminally ill', *Journal of Hospice Palliative Nursing*, 9(3): 159–67.

Koffman, J. and Higginson, I.J. (2001) 'Accounts of carers' satisfaction with health care at the end of life: a comparison of first generation black Caribbeans and white patients with advanced disease', *Palliative Medicine*, 15: 337–45.

Life as a House (2001) Irwin Winkler (Director). Winkler Films, USA.

McGinn, M. (2010) *End of Life Care Module*. South West London Cancer Network [online]. Available at: www.onlinecancereducationforum.com/OCEF/Endoflifecare. pdfEn [accessed 11 September 2012].

Meghani, S. (2003) 'A concept analysis of palliative care in the United States', *Journal of Advanced Nursing*, 46(2): 152–61.

National Council for Palliative Care (NCPC) (2006) *Changing Gear: Guidelines for Managing the Last Days of Life in Adults*. London: NCPC.

National Council for Palliative Care (NCPC) (2012) *Dying Matters* [online]. Available at: www.dyingmatters.org [accessed 11 September 2012].

National Gold Standards Framework Centre (2012) [online]. Available at: www.goldstandards framework.org.uk [accessed 11 September 2012].

NICE (National Institute for Health and Clinical Excellence) (2004) *Improving Supportive and Palliative Care for Adults with Cancer* London: National Institute for Clinical Excellence.

Office for National Statistics (1998) *1996 Mortality Statistics*. General Series DH No. 28. London: HMSO.

Oxford Dictionary (2012) [online]. Available at: www.oxforddictionaries.com/definition/palliative [accessed 11 September 2012].

Philadelphia (1993) Jonathan Demme (Director). ClinicaEstetico, USA.

Seymour, J., Clark, D. and Winslow, M. (2005) 'Pain and palliative care: the emergence of new specialties', *Journal of Pain and Symptom Management*, 29(1): 2–13.

Stjernsward, J. and Clark, D. (2004) 'Palliative medicine a global perspective', in D. Doyle, G. Hanks, N. Cherry and K. Calman (eds), *Oxford Textbook of Palliative Medicine* (3rd edn). Oxford: Oxford University Press.

The Bucket List (2007) Ron Reiner (Director). Warner Bros., USA.

Tothill, M. (1999) *Little Company of Mary Sisters: Early Beginnings* [online]. Available at: www.lcmsisters.org.uk/EarlyBeginnings.html [accessed 11 September 2012].

Trueman, I. and Parker, J. (2006) 'Exploring community nurses' perceptions of life review in palliative care', *Journal of Clinical Nursing*, 15: 197–207.

WHO (2006) 'World Health Organisation pain and palliative care communication program: appraising the WHO analgesic ladder on its 20th anniversary', *Cancer Pain Release*, 19(1). Available at: www.whocancerpain.wisc.edu/index?q=node/86 [accessed 11 September 2012].

WHO (2012) World Health Organisation Definition of Palliative Care [online]. Available at: www.who.int/cancer/palliative/definition/en/ [accessed 11 September 2012].

CHAPTER 2

Assessing holistic needs

Annie Pettifer

This chapter will explore:

- Holistic needs assessment
- The tools that are available to support holistic assessment
- How to structure an assessment conversation

Holistic needs assessment

The significance of assessment runs deep in palliative and end-of-life care, as thorough holistic assessment of patients is key to the provision of good end-of-life care.

Assessment is the first step in determining the health needs of any patient. Its importance in end-of-life care is paramount which is emphasised in key documents. For example, Chapter 1 described the World Health Organisation's seminal definition of palliative and end-of-life care (WHO 2012), which includes 'impeccable assessment'. Within the End of Life Care Strategy (Department of Health 2008), assessment is the second element of the end-of-life care pathway.

Assessment provides an important opportunity to establish a therapeutic relationship within which patients can talk through and clarify their preferences with a health professional. Potentially it provides the opportunity for unmet needs and concerns to be identified and shared. Appropriate ongoing care, centred around patients' preferences and needs, can be agreed, planned and then shared appropriately. Sharing assessment and the resulting care plans with others may result in the need for fewer individual assessments by individual health and social care providers. If all are working collaboratively from one assessment and plan, care is likely to be more consistent and repetitious conversations can be avoided.

The word 'holistic' originates from the Greek word for whole and as such infers consideration of a patient as a whole person with many facets and needs, including psychological, social, spiritual, emotional and physical needs. Each of these should be considered.

The significance of holistic assessment can be seen in the following comment by a patient to Dame Cicely Saunders in her early career:

> Well... it [pain] began in my back, but now it seems that all of me is wrong. ... I could have cried for the pills and the injections, but I knew that I mustn't. The world seemed to be against me, nobody seemed to understand how I felt. My husband and son were marvellous, but they were having to stay off work and lose their money.
>
> (Mrs Hinton to Cicely Saunders [online], available at: http://commtechlab.msu.edu/ sites/cancerpain/CicelySaunders/CS_Aindex.htm)

From this quotation, it is evident that Mrs Hinton's pain is far more complex than simply a physical experience, and that to understand it requires an assessment of her psychological, social, spiritual, emotional and physical needs or domains. Simply treating her physical sensation would have limited impact on her pain.

The following case study provides a context for a holistic assessment with a patient, Mr Clarkson, who has some complex needs. Threaded throughout this chapter, it raises principles and highlights information and the tools required to develop good needs assessment skills.

Mr Clarkson

John, a third-year student nurse in a community placement, attended a multidisciplinary team meeting held in a community health centre at which his mentor, Sue, a district nurse, presented a gentleman called Dave Clarkson.

Mr Clarkson, aged 47, had been troubled by painful swallowing (dysphagia) and indigestion for some time but delayed seeking medical advice until some weeks after the symptoms started. At that stage both eating solid and liquid foods had become painful. A barium swallow showed a large lesion in the mid-oesophagus which, following endoscopic biopsy, was found to be a squamous cell carcinoma. Staging investigations, including Computerised Tomography (CT) and Position Emission Tomography (PET) scans, showed a spread to the surrounding lymph nodes and lung metastases. Mr

(Continued)

CASE STUDY

(Continued)

Clarkson had palliative radiotherapy, chemotheraphy and stenting which improved his swallowing for some weeks. Recently, however, the problem has increased, alongside progressive weakness and weight loss. He has also been coughing up small amounts of blood (hemoptysis).

Mr Clarkson has a history of high alcohol use and smokes around 30 cigarettes a day. He also has a history of depression. He is currently living in hostel accommodation. He has a sister but lost touch with her some time ago. He is aware of his diagnosis but has asked few questions about his future. He is reluctant to accept day care in the local hospice or to have a Macmillan nurse visit him at home. However, he does attend follow-up appointments in the local outpatients department and is willing to see a specialist there. Sue recommends holistic assessment within a nurse-led clinic at outpatients. Following discussion, Farah the specialist palliative care nurse, agrees to do this.

John asks to attend this assessment in the following week, wondering how Mr Clarkson's complex needs will be assessed.

Action point

Consider what Mr Clarkson's psychological, social, spiritual, emotional and physical needs (domains) might be.

Mr Clarkson's needs are clearly complex and span all the domains mentioned above. They may include the need for appropriate housing. Physical symptoms are evident. Given his depression, he may be particularly vulnerable, and it will be important to assess the extent of this. He may or may not wish to re-establish contact with his family. He may well have questions and worries that he has not yet spoken of.

The End of Life Care Programme recommends that all patients approaching the end of their lives should be offered a holistic assessment (National End of Life Care Programme 2010a). Assessment *per se* is part and parcel of ongoing care, and is not limited to particular interactions focused on assessment. However, ideally patients should be offered focused holistic assessment when

- the end-of-life phase is identified,
- when it is evident they are dying,
- when requested by the individual patient, or
- when judged necessary by a professional (National End of Life Care Programme 2010a).

In Mr Clarkson's case, holistic assessment has been recommended by his district nurse.

A member of the caring team should undertake holistic assessment. Clearly they must have the appropriate assessment skills and knowledge required (National End of Life

Care Programme 2010a). Patients' preferences for assessment should be respected and, in Mr Clarkson's case, a venue has been arranged that ensures he is not assessed in a hospice setting.

The tools that are available to support holistic assessment

The National End of Life Care Programme (2010a) encourages health and social care providers to develop a shared common holistic assessment, including appropriate assessment tools. The programme does not in itself advocate specific holistic tools, but gives advice on how such tools might be developed. It recommends dividing the assessment into five domains that should be covered within a conversation. These are:

- Background information and assessment preferences
- Physical needs
- Social and occupational needs
- Psychological well-being
- Spiritual well-being and life goals.

While there is a paucity of published validated tools for comprehensive holistic assessment, a number of useful tools which assess a limited range of needs are available. These include the Sheffield Profile for Assessment and Referral to Care (SPARC), the Northern Ireland Single Assessment Tool, and the PEPSI COLA *aide-mémoire* (National End of Life Care Programme 2010a). While these all have their limitations, they can provide a useful framework to structure a holistic assessment. In addition, a number of tools focus on the assessment of specific aspects of care, such as depression (Lloyd-Williams et al. 2000) or spiritual care (Anandarajah and Hight 2001). While these tools may be useful, they differ from holistic assessment tools since they are confined to one aspect of care.

Two assessment tools that consider a range of needs are described briefly below.

PEPSI COLA *aide-mémoire*

This tool was designed for use within the Gold Standards Framework (Gold Standards Framework Centre 2009) and has been widely endorsed (National End of Life Care Programme 2010a; National Cancer Action Team 2012). It is an *aide-mémoire* for considering holistic domains and uses the following acronym:

P – Physical

E – Emotional

P – Personal

S – Social support

I – Information and communication

C – Control

O – Out of hours

L – Late (on some versions this is 'Living with your illness')

A – Aftercare

Each of the headings triggered from the acronym are expanded to prompt the assessor to consider exploring that domain or aspect of a patient in some detail. For example, within the 'emotional' domain, the tool prompts 'psychological assessment' including the expectations of the patient, their mood, relationships with others, and fears and anxieties. Such prompts are simply to assist practitioners and should be used with careful consideration rather than by rote. It may be that some prompts are not relevant at some times or to some patients. Having considered what needs are to be assessed, the PEPSI COLA *aide-mémoire* gives examples of helpful cues and questions that may assist practitioners in making assessments. For example, a suggested cue question to assess emotional domain is *'what is worrying you most?'* Finally, the *aide-mémoire* offers a list of relevant resources on which practitioners may draw. For example, under the emotional domain, a suggested resource is the 'distress thermometer'.

Sheffield Profile for Assessment and Referral to Care (SPARC)

SPARC was developed by the Academic Unit of Supportive Care at Sheffield University to identify patients who should be referred to specialist palliative care (Ahmedzai et al. 2004). It is a questionnaire that can be posted to patients prior to assessment. Within the questionnaire are 45 questions covering:

- Communication and information issues
- Physical symptoms
- Psychological issues
- Religious and spiritual issues
- Independence and activity
- Family and social issues
- Treatment issues
- Personal issues

Patients are mostly asked to rate the questions on a four-point scale to indicate the level of distress they have experienced in these areas. For some questions this scale is inappropriate, and patients are just asked to give a 'yes' or 'no' response.

Assessment tools can be adapted for local use by health care organisations and individual practitioners. All have their advantages and disadvantages, and all have a different emphasis (Richardson et al. 2007). The Association for Palliative Medicine Clinical Effectiveness Group has produced the 'Which Tool?' Guide (Association for Palliative Medicine of Great Britain and Ireland 2001), which offers some evaluation of the assessment tools available, and further evaluation is available in the holistic common assessment guidance section of the National End of Life Care Programme (2010a).

> ## Action point
>
> When you are next in practice, find out which holistic assessment tools are used in your area.

When thinking about which tool may best help us to assess Mr Clarkson it might be helpful to consider the following. Mr Clarkson has been referred for a holistic assessment and has complex needs spanning a number of domains. Therefore, the initial assessment tool needs to be comprehensive. The primary purpose of this assessment is clinical rather than research-focused, and therefore the tool needs to be appropriate for this purpose. The assessment will take place in a clinic setting where there may be considerable time constraints. Therefore the tool must not be overly lengthy or laborious.

The PEPSI COLA *aide-mémoire* is appropriate and likely to be useful for assessing Mr Clarkson. It is a practice-centred tool which can be used simply to guide the practitioner through the process of assessment, ensuring that all domains have been considered. It suggests a way that aspects of these domains may be assessed through conversation, particularly the use of cue questions, issue-specific assessment tools and additional resources.

How to structure an assessment conversation

A holistic assessment is in essence a conversation in which health professionals offer patients an opportunity to express their concerns and to be listened to actively. It is inherently dependent on good communication skills, particularly those of sensitively eliciting concerns, actively listening to the response and negotiating a care plan in which the patient's concerns and needs are central.

In the case study, John wonders how Farah will go about holistically assessing Mr Clarkson's needs. This section will consider in some detail how Farah might go about this, as an example of holistic assessment per se.

The Cambridge–Calgary Consultation Model (Silverman et al. 2005) gives helpful guidance for structuring consultations between health care practitioners and patients. It includes assessment discussions using five key headings and two themes, which must be kept in mind throughout the conversation. This model will assist the assessment of Mr Clarkson's needs.

Initiating the session

In this crucial phase Farah needs quickly to establish an initial rapport with Mr Clarkson through greeting him, introducing herself and any others present, such as John, and explaining their various roles. Farah needs to make clear the purpose of the impending conversation, so that Mr Clarkson knows what to expect. Research by Heaven and Maguire (1997) into hospice patients' disclosure of their concerns to nurses, demonstrates that patients tailor the information they disclose according to their expectations of the role and purpose of the person asking. Therefore it is important that Farah defines her role and purpose effectively. She could consider saying something like:

> Hello Mr Clarkson. My name is Farah Abbas. I am a specialist nurse from the hospice. Sue asked me to see you here today as I understand you have some health problems which I may be able to help with.

Through these early greetings, Farah needs to convey her interest in Mr Clarkson and her willingness to hear his concerns. While there is no one way of doing this, sitting down, making eye contact and leaning slightly forward are all ways of showing interest. Sometimes, briefly asking something conversational, such as about their travel to the clinic, or commenting on the weather, can help put people at their ease.

Gathering information

The second step of the Cambridge–Calgary Consultation Model is gathering information (Silverman et al. 2005).

Part of an assessment involves gathering information that is already known. Full referral information is vital to give a detailed picture of the patient's circumstances. Existing relevant health and social records should be studied to ensure assessors are familiar with the patient's history and treatment. Additional information may be gathered from talking to recent carers.

Farah has already gained information about Mr Clarkson from the multidisciplinary meeting in which he was discussed. Farah is likely to have access to electronic and paper records in the hospital clinic, and she may also wish to speak to hostel staff to gain information about Mr Clarkson's current situation.

Within the actual consultation, Farah needs to fully explore Mr Clarkson's problems from his own perspective by inviting him to tell her about his concerns.

Reflective question

The following four statements are ways that Farah might invite Mr Clarkson to talk about his concerns. Which do you imagine Mr Clarkson might find most helpful?

1 I have been asked by ... to assess your needs holistically. Please can you tell me what they are?
2 How are things for you at the moment?
3 I understand you have not been well recently. Would you tell me what happened please?
4 The first thing on my list is physical. How are you physically?

There is no right or wrong way to invite a patient to talk about his/her concerns. Everyone has different styles and language. However, there are key principles that may help clarify which approaches may be most helpful. Although question 2 directly asks Mr Clarkson to think about how he is now, it is predominantly an open question as it leaves Mr Clarkson able to answer in almost any way he chooses. This may be helpful to some patients, but may also be baffling if someone is unsure what response is expected. In this case it may only precipitate a short response such as 'all right'.

Questions 1 and 4 are both much more direct. Question 1 is very clear, but the word 'holistic' may be unfamiliar to those outside health care. The question does not convey warmth or concern. Question 4 is even more direct and perfunctory. It does not give scope for Mr Clarkson to voice non-physical concerns. Question 3 is an open direct question that can be responded to in a number of ways, but gives some focus as to where to start. When delivered in a caring manner it would imply empathy and a willingness to listen. It invites Mr Clarkson to tell his story of his illness....

Farah: I understand you have not been well recently. Would you tell me what happened please?

Mr Clarkson: It just hurt when I ate. Didn't mind much ... bound to I suppose, but when it got to this state it was no good. Had some needles and rays and stuff at the hospital, don't think it did much. Gets me right down. I'm in my boots. Why did it have to come now, just when I was finding my feet?

Here we can see how Farah's question has enabled Mr Clarkson to tell her something of his story. His answer gives useful clues about his concerns, and is therefore a starting point for assessing them in detail. Importantly, this approach is patient-focused as opposed to focused on the agenda of his health care practitioner.

> ## Action point
>
> When observing assessments, as John is doing in this case, notice how practitioners initiate assessment conversations. Try to remember phrases that seem helpful and that you might use in future.

The Cambridge–Calgary Model prompts gathering information relating to domains, in much the same way as the PEPSI COLA *aide-mémoire* does. This is the stage of the conversation where the acronym can be used to ensure that the concerns Mr Clarkson has raised are explored in some detail and that all relevant domains have been assessed.

All domains covered by the PEPSI COLA *aide-mémoire* will need to be considered, although some may not be relevant and therefore Farah may decide not to raise them with Mr Clarkson, or delay discussing them until a subsequent meeting. The emotional, personal and control domains are particularly relevant to Mr Clarkson's case and will therefore be discussed in detail below as examples. Assessment of common physical symptoms at the end of life is considered in Chapter 6. Table 2.1 at the end of this chapter shows a possible assessment strategy, cue questions and tools using PEPSI COLA *aide-mémoire*. It is not designed to be comprehensive, but illustrates how the PEPSI COLA *aide-mémoire* may be used.

'E' – The emotional domain

The emotional domain prompts psychological assessment, including the expectations of the patients, their wishes for information, and their mood, fears and anxieties. Mr Clarkson's response, 'It gets me right down. I'm down in my boots', indicates the need to explore his psychological needs in some depth. He appears to have low expectations of the treatment he has had and his mood is also low.

The term 'distress' is used to encompass psychological needs. Thekkumpurath et al. (2008) consider the concept of distress in people who are at the end of their lives. They use the following definition from the National Comprehensive Cancer Network (2007):

> a multifactorial unpleasant emotional experience of a psychological (cognitive, behavioural, or emotional), social, and/or spiritual nature. ... Distress extends along a continuum from common normal feelings of vulnerability and sadness ... to problems that can become disabling, such as depression, anxiety, panic, social isolation, and existential and spiritual crisis. (Thekkumpurath et al. 2008: 520)

The definition demonstrates the scope of distress that Mr Clarkson may be experiencing and infers the need to explore the point he has reached along the continuum.

Distress is common among people at the end of their lives. While estimates vary according to the way in which they are derived, research suggests that up to 50% of people with advanced cancer and poor prognosis experience distress (Hotopf et al. 2002) and that much of it is not detected by health practitioners (Thekkumpurath et al. 2008). This is partly through patients normalising it or simply putting up with it as an expected part of being so ill, and partly due to lack of good assessment. However, if successfully recognised, distress can be improved through a range of interventions, including medications and psychological support.

Assessing Mr Clarkson's emotional needs requires great sensitivity. Farah may consider the history of Mr Clarkson's low mood and to what extent it relates or pre-dates his current problems. She will need a description of his low moods, including their severity, together with their impact both on him and on those around him. It will be important to consider how he copes, and the effect of any medication or psychological interventions that have been tried (National End of Life Care Programme 2010a).

The PEPSI COLA *aide-mémoire* suggests possible cue questions which might be useful in this assessment, such as 'How do you normally cope in stressful situations?' It also suggests the use of structured screening tools. One such tool that focuses on distress is the Edinburgh Depression Scale (Cox et al. 1987). This tool was originally devised to assess new mothers. It asks patients to rate 10 statements relating to their mood on a 4-point scale. For example, the first statement is: 'I have been able to laugh and see the funny side of things'.

The Edinburgh Depression Scale has been validated in inpatient and day centre patients with advanced cancer (Lloyd-Williams et al. 2000; Lloyd-Williams et al. 2004).

Reflective question

If you were in Farah's shoes, how would you begin a conversation to assess Mr Clarkson's emotional needs? You may consider the following three suggestions or think of another approach of your own.

1 Ask him to complete the Edinburgh Depression Scale.
2 Ask him – 'Are you depressed at the moment?'
3 Following on from the conversation given above, ask him to say a little more about his mood.

When considering how best to assess Mr Clarkson's emotional needs it is important to bear in mind the roles of the various health care practitioners. The National Institute of Clinical Excellence (NICE) (2004) describes levels of professional psychological assessment and support. At level one, all health and social care professionals should be able to 'recognise psychological needs'. At this level, using a recognised assessment tool is optional (End of Life Care Programme 2010a). However, as a nurse specialist in palliative care, Farah has additional expertise and therefore her role includes screening for psychological distress. She may consider a tool to do this.

Farah could start by picking up from Mr Clarkson's earlier response. She might say something like:

> *Farah*: I am sorry to hear you are so down at the moment. Can you tell me a bit more about that?

This question aims to acknowledge what he has said, show some concern about it, and invite him to tell Farah some more. While the question 'Are you depressed?' may be helpful, its usefulness is variable (Thekkumpurath et al. 2008). At this stage it may be too blunt and may not demonstrate empathy or listening. Structured screening tools also have their problems. They can be laborious for sick patients to complete. Rates of illiteracy are higher than average among homeless people (Olisa et al. 2010) and it may be that Mr Clarkson would not choose to complete a form even with assistance.

'P' – The personal domain

The personal domain considers specific personal needs such as those derived from culture or ethnicity, language, sexuality and spirituality. In Mr Clarkson's case, issues of spirituality are pertinent. His comment '*Why does it have to come now?*' is worthy of further exploration. It may indicate a spiritual need.

The Department of Health commissioned a systematic review of spiritual care (Universities of Hull, Staffordshire and Aberdeen 2011) to support the End of Life Care Strategy (Department of Health 2008). While this report acknowledges the complexity of defining the concept of spirituality, it offers the following parameters:

> Spirituality relates to the way in which people understand and live their lives in view of their core beliefs and values, and their perception of ultimate meaning. Spirituality includes the need to find satisfactory answers to ultimate questions about the meaning of life, illness and death. (Universities of Hull, Staffordshire and Aberdeen 2011: 18)

Mr Clarkson may be struggling to make sense of his advancing illness and impending death. The question of why the end of his life is approaching now is profoundly difficult and raises spiritual dilemmas. It is not unusual that Mr Clarkson's thoughts are turning to existential questions. As people approach the end of their lives many will wonder what the meaning or purpose of their life has been. They may review important relationships such as that with their parents or children. For some, such thoughts may be framed through a religious faith, for others it may be more secular.

Wright (2004) writes that spirituality encompasses the following aspects of human beings:

- Personhood – this can be seen in the values and beliefs held by the person that shape the way he or she lives
- Relationships – with self, others, life force/God/universe/spirit
- Search for meaning – in life and death
- Transcendence – belief in something beyond ourselves
- Religion – prayer, communion, vocation and worship

Spiritual assessment once again demands great sensitivity. A number of structured spiritual tools have been devised (Anandarajah and Hight 2001; Narayanasamy 2004). However, the validity of such tools is unclear (Universities of Hull, Staffordshire and Aberdeen 2011). Rather than attempting to quantify such complex human questions, it may be better just to listen actively to patients who wish to discuss such concerns without judging them in any way.

The following example shows how Farah might do this:

Mr Clarkson: Why did it have to happen, I was just finding my feet?

Farah: You are wondering why this has happened to you.

Farah's question is purposefully phrased as a sentence. It makes no comment but invites Mr Clarkson to say more if he wishes. He may choose to answer:

Mr Clarkson: Yeah, Just doesn't make sense does it – talk about kicking a man when he is down. When I was a kid, my Mum said that, you know – him up there took care of you. So much for that.

This response raises many more spiritual issues. Mr Clarkson is expressing the unfairness of his situation and shows concern for the incongruence between this and his childhood view. He also raises transcendence, or a belief in something beyond humankind.

'C' – The control domain

The control domain is concerned with discussions of patient choices and advance care planning.

Advance care planning (ACP) is central to the provision of appropriate and seamless care outside normal working hours. Advance care planning is the proactive advance care planning through discussion between a patient and health care professional to consider and document the patient's wishes for their future care (National End of Life Care Programme 2008). There is no standard form for documenting advance care plans and many care organisations have developed their own. An example of this is 'Planning Ahead', devised by Weston Hospice Care, which draws together legally valid forms in which patients can document their wishes for future care. (See Further reading for website.)

Advance care planning is voluntary and should not be undertaken routinely as a part of general care (National End of Life Care Programme 2008). However, it may be that some discussion of Mr Clarkson's wishes has already been undertaken, perhaps by hostel staff who know him well. It may appropriate to offer Mr Clarkson the opportunity to discuss his wishes, either within the assessment or at another time.

Below are two examples of how Farah might initiate this discussion:

> *Farah*: Sue told me that you particularly wanted to meet me here. Do you have any other preferences about your care?

> *Farah*: Some people in your situation like to talk through how they want to be looked after, and what they want professionals to do or not do. I wonder if you have had the chance to do that with anyone?

This section has considered three of the PEPSI COLA *aide-mémoire* domains that are particularly relevant to the holistic assessment of Mr Clarkson. Suggestions for the full assessment of Mr Clarkson, considering all the domains within the PEPSI COLA *aide-mémoire* are given in Figure 2.1 at the end of this chapter.

Physical examination

The Cambridge–Calgary Consultation Model includes considering physical examination at this point. The purpose of physical examination at the end of life should be to glean information that can be used to enhance comfort. Therefore it may or may not be applicable.

Explanation and planning

The structure of the Cambridge–Calgary consultation emphasises the importance of deferring planning of care until after all the information has been gathered. It may be helpful to acknowledge the problems and concerns that have been raised in the assessment with a brief summary. Once again it is important to check that the assessment is accurate. Farah could achieve this by sharing her documentation of the assessment with Mr Clarkson and asking him whether it is accurate. Alternatively, she could summarise it verbally. For example, she might say:

> *Farah*: You clearly have a lot on your mind at the moment. It is difficult to swallow your food. You are feeling weak and worried that you have lost so much weight. There are spots of blood coming up when you cough sometimes. Have I got that right?

It is important to check that Mr Clarkson has been able to voice all his concerns. For example:

> *Farah*: Is there anything else troubling you?

He may wish to ask questions about his care or the assessment process.

Care planning should be a collaborative process between the patient and the assessor. It is important to bear in mind that what patients want may not always be predictable by professionals. Health care professionals should discuss what the management options are and what is realistically achievable. Where there are a number of problems it might be helpful to prioritise them, so that care planning can address them accordingly. For example:

> *Farah*: From what you have said, the worst thing for you at the moment is the worry about where you will be living in the future. Is that also the most urgent thing for you now?

Closing the session

Clearly, patients may wish to discuss what may happen to the assessment, how it will be used and with whom it will be shared. They may also wish to have a copy of the documentation.

Summary

The key points to remember when undertaking holistic assessment are:

- Holistic assessments are an opportunity for patients and health or social care professionals to discuss patients' concerns and preferences for future care.
- Holistic assessments are a comprehensive consideration of a patient's situation.
- While assessment tools can be useful, a holistic assessment is essentially a conversation and relies on good communication skills.

Further reading

Milligan's article is an excellent starting point for learning more about spiritual care. Part of the *Nursing Standard*'s 'Learning Zone' series, it details spiritual care in an accessible way:

Milligan, S. (2011) 'Addressing the spiritual care needs of people near the end of life', *Nursing Standard*, 26(4): 47–56.

Pearce and Duffy's chapter on holistic care gives further detail about this subject:

Pearce, C.M. and Duffy, A. (2005) 'Holistic care', Chapter 3 in J. Lugton and R. McIntyre (eds), *Palliative Care the Nursing Role* (2nd edn). Oxford: Elsevier.

Taylor and Ashelford's article is also part of the 'Learning Zone' series but addresses the subject of depression:

Taylor, V. and Ashelford, S. (2008) 'Understanding depression in palliative and end of life care', *Nursing Standard*, 23(12): 48–57.

An online link to the Cambridge–Calgary Consultation Model can be found at: www. skillscascade.com/handouts/CalgaryCambridgeGuide.pdf.

A number of versions of the PEPSI COLA *aide-mémoire* can be found online, including the two below:

www.cwdgp.org.au/page/Services/Programs/Palliative_Care/Palliative_Care_Templates_and_ Tools [accessed 4 May 2012]

www.goldstandardsframework.nhs.uk/OneStopCMS/Core/CrawlerResourceServer. aspx?resource=2E9DA6B2-5D8D-4D3B-8315-C0FA90181045 [accessed 5 May 2012]

An example of an advanced care plan can be found at Weston Hospice Care:

www.westonhospicecaregroup.org.uk/patients-families/end-of-life-registeradvanced-care-planning/ [accessed 4 May 2012]

References

Ahmedzai, S.H., Payne, S.A., Bestall, J.C., Ahmed, N., Dobson, K., Clark, D. et al. (2004) *Improving Access to Specialist Palliative Care: Developing a Screening Measure to Assess the Distress Caused by Advanced Illness that May Require Referral to Specialist Palliative Care*. Sheffield: University of Sheffield and Trent Palliative Care Centre, 42.

Anandarajah, G. and Hight, E. (2001) 'Spirituality and medical practice: using HOPE questions as a practical tool for spiritual assessment', *American Family Physician*, 63(1): 81–9.

Association for Palliative Medicine of Great Britain and Ireland (Clinical Effectiveness Group) (2001) *The 'Which Tool' Guide: Preliminary Review of Tools to Measure Clinical Effectiveness in Palliative Care*. Association for Palliative Medicine of Great Britain and Ireland [online]. Available at: www.palliative-medicine.org/resources/images/Whichtoolguide.doc [accessed 4 May 2012].

Cox, J.L., Holden, J.M. and Sagovsky, R. (1987) 'Detection of postnatal depression: development of the 10-item Edinburgh Postnatal Depression Scale', *British Journal of Psychiatry*, 150: 782–6.

Department of Health (2008) *The End of Life Care Strategy: Promoting High Quality Care for All Adults at the End of Life, Equality Impact Assessment*. London: Department of Health.

Gold Standards Framework Centre (2009) *The PEPSI COLA Aide-mémoire* [online]. Available at: www.goldstandardsframework.nhs.uk/OneStopCMS/Core/CrawlerResourceServer.aspx? resource=2E9DA6B2-5D8D-4D3B-8315-C0FA90181045 [accessed 4 May 2012].

Heaven, C.M. and Maguire, P. (1997) 'Disclosure of concerns by hospice patients and their identification by nurses', *Palliative Medicine*, 4: 283–90.

Hotopf, M., Chidgey, J., Addington-Hall, J. and Ly, K.L. (2002) 'Depression in advanced disease: a systematic review. Part 1: Prevalence and case finding', *Palliative Medicine*, 16: 81–97.

Lloyd-Williams, M., Dennis, M. and Taylor, F. (2004) 'A prospective study to compare three depression screening tools in patients who are terminally ill', *General Hospital Psychiatry*, 26: 384–9.

Lloyd-Williams, M., Friedman, T. and Rudd, N. (2000) 'Criterion validation of Edinburgh Post Natal Depression Scale as a screening tool for depression in patients with metastatic advanced metastatic cancer', *Journal of Pain and Symptom Management*, 20: 259–65.

Narayanasamy, A. (2004) 'The puzzle of spirituality for nursing: a guide to practical assessment', *British Journal of Nursing*, 13(19): 1140–4.

National Cancer Action Team (2012) *Holistic Needs Assessment for People with Cancer: A Practical Guide for Health Care Professionals* [online]. Available at: http://ncat.nhs.uk/sites/default/files/HNA_practical%20guide_web.pdf [accessed 5 May 2012].

National Comprehensive Cancer Network (2007) 'Clinical practice guidelines in oncology', cited in Thekkumpurath, P., Venkataswaran, C., Kumar, M. and Bennett, M. (2008) 'Screening or psychological distress in palliative care: a systematic review', *Journal of Pain and Symptom Management*, 36(5): 520–8.

National End of Life Care Programme (2008) *Advance Care Planning: Guide for Health and Social Care Staff* [online]. Available at: www.endoflifecareforadults.nhs.uk/assets/downloads/pubs_Advance_Care_Planning_guide.pdf [accessed 24 April 2012].

National End of Life Care Programme (2010a) *Holistic Common Assessment of Supportive and Palliative Care Needs for Adults Requiring End of Life Care* [online]. Available at: www.endoflifecareforadults.nhs.uk/assets/downloads/HCA_guide.pdf [accessed 14 March 2012].

National End of Life Care Programme (2010b) *End of Life Care: Achieving Quality in Hostels and for Homeless People – A Route to Success* [online]. Available at: www.endoflifecareforadults.nhs.uk/assets/downloads/RTS_Homeless_Final_draft_20101211.pdf [accessed 5 May 2012].

National Institute for Clinical Excellence (2004) *Improving Supportive and Palliative Care for Adults with Cancer* [online]. Available at: www.nice.org.uk/nicemedia/live/10893/28816/28816.pdf [accessed 30 March 2012].

Olisa, J., Patterson, J. and Wright, F. (2010) *Turning the Key: Portraits of Low Literacy amongst People with Experience of Homelessness. Thames Reach* [online]. Available at: www.thamesreach.org.uk/publications/research-reports/turning-the-key/ [accessed 4 May 2012].

Richardson, A., Medina, J., Brown, V. and Sitzia, J. (2007) 'Patients' needs assessment in cancer care: a review of assessment tools', *Supportive Care in Cancer*, 15: 1125–44.

Silverman, J.D., Kurtz, S.M. and Draper, J. (2005) *Skills for Communicating with Patients* (2nd edn). Oxford: Radcliffe Publishing.

Thekkumpurath, P., Venkataswaran, C., Kumar, M. and Bennett, M. (2008) 'Screening or psychological distress in palliative care: a systematic review', *Journal of Pain and Symptom Management*, 36(5): 520–8.

Universities of Hull, Staffordshire and Aberdeen (2011) *Spiritual Care at the End of Life: A Systematic Review of the Literature* [online]. London: Department of Health. Available at: www.dh.gov.uk/prod_consum_dh/groups/dh_digitalassets/@dh/@en/documents/digitalasset/dh_123804.pdf [accessed 7 May 2012].

WHO (2012) World Health Organisation Definition of Palliative Care [online]. Available at: www.who.int/cancer/palliative/definition/en/ [accessed 5 May 2012].

Wright, M.C. (2004) 'Good for the soul?', Chapter 11 in S. Payne, J. Seymour and C. Ingleton (eds), *Palliative Care Nursing: Principles and Evidence for Practice*. Buckingham: Open University Press.

Table 2.1   Possible assessment strategy, cue questions and tools using PEPSI COLA *aide-mémoire*

This Table gives suggestions of how each area of the PEPSI COLA *aide-mémoire* may be used to assess Mr Clarkson's holistic needs. It is intended as a guide and not to be used verbatim. While assessment of all areas should be considered by assessors, they need to select which areas are relevant. For example, it may not be appropriate to raise issues surrounding terminal care and bereavement issues at this stage, as prompted within the 'late' and 'aftercare' domains.

Furthermore, patient-centred assessment focuses on inviting patients to tell their story rather than complete a series of questions. In this context, questions should be used to ensure that all relevant areas have been considered. However, assessors need to be mindful of the burden that asking multiple questions can have on sick patients and modify their assessment accordingly.

PEPSI COLA domain	Problem/issue identified	Assessment strategy, cue questions and tools

PHYSICAL	Dysphagia (painful swallowing)	Take a history of dysphagia
		
		Ask questions like:
		  Duration – How long have you had it?
		  Descriptions – Please describe what happens when you swallow. What does the pain feel like?
		
		Severity – How difficult is it? What types of food and drink are most difficult?
		Impact – How is this affecting you? How much weight have you lost? Are you hungry? Is it affecting the way you eat with others?
		Intervention – What, if any, medication are you taking, in what dose and how often?
		Relief – What makes it better or worse?
		
		Consider specialist speech and language therapy assessment.

	Hemoptysis (coughing up blood)	Take a history of hemoptysis
		
		Ask questions like:
		  Duration – How long have you noticed blood when you cough?
		  Severity – how often does this happen? How much blood is there?
		  Impact – does this worry you?
		  Intervention – Are you taking any medication for it?
		
		Observe for volume of blood and frequency while with patients. What effect is this having on your daily activities?
		
		Observe for signs of possible infection, e.g. pyrexia.

(Continued)

PEPSI COLA domain	Problem/issue identified	Assessment strategy, cue questions and tools
EMOTIONAL	Low mood	Ask questions like: What worries you most at the moment? How do you normally cope in stressful situations? How has your mood been in the past? Screen for depression – e.g. Do you feel agitated, irritable, hopeless, guilty, worthlessness? Do you have low self-esteem? Are you socially withdrawn? Consider using depression screening tool such as Edinburgh Depression Scale (Cox et al. 1987).
PERSONAL	Spiritual issues	Ask questions like: How do you make sense of what is happening to you? Or is there anything you would like us to do to respect your religious needs? Consider using a spiritual assessment tool such as Narayanasamy (2004). Do you have any particular religious beliefs? Consider whether referral is needed – e.g. Would you find it helpful to talk to someone who could help you explore the issues?
SOCIAL	Family and social situation	Consider Mr Clarkson's current housing situation. Liaise with hostel staff to assess challenges of caring for someone at the end of their lives in a hostel setting – both for staff and for other residents (National End of Life Care Programme 2010b) Consider whether Mr Clarkson would like to re-establish contact with his sister.
INFORMATION	Access to appropriate information	Ask questions like: Do you know how to contact services to help you at this time, e.g. GP, district nurses? Do you have any questions about how and when to contact different services, and whom to ask for? Is there any additional information that you require?
CONTROL	Loss of control/ advanced care planning	Consider preferences for care. Ask questions like: Have you discussed and documented your future care with anyone? Have you written down your wishes? If yes, where is it kept? Where would you like to be cared for in the next few days? Who would you like to care for you in the next few days?

(Continued)

Table 2.1   (Continued)

PEPSI COLA domain	Problem/issue identified	Assessment strategy, cue questions and tools
OUT OF HOURS	Care outside normal working hours	Ask questions like: Are you aware of who to call for out-of-hours advice and assistance? Do you and the hostel staff know how to contact service(s) out of hours, or if there is an emergency.
LATE	Terminal care	Ask questions like: Do you have any other symptoms that you are concerned about? Do you have any concerns/anxieties about the next 24/48 hours?
AFTERCARE	Bereavement issues	Ask questions like: Is there anything more you want to say/ information you want us to have? Are there any affairs you wish to attend to?

Adapted from PEPSI COLA *aide-mémoire*

CHAPTER 3

Responding to questions about the end of life

Annie Pettifer

This chapter will explore:

- Why good communication matters
- Blocking and facilitating communication strategies
- Why health care professionals block communication with dying patients and their families
- Who should respond to difficult questions?
- Breaking bad news sensitively
- Sources of support for students

Introduction

Communication between nurses and patients arguably forms the foundation of all health care. It is the interaction between two or more people that conveys meaningful information between them. Sensitive and skilled communication is particularly key to caring for patients who are facing the end of their lives. Therefore, mastery of this interaction by health care professionals will enhance the end-of-life care hugely. This chapter focuses on communication in end-of-life care covering the crucial areas of assessing patients' concerns, handling difficult questions and breaking bad news. The following case study of Mary, a woman contemplating the end of her life, and Rosie, the student caring for her, raises a challenging situation of how to respond to a very difficult question – whether or not a person is going to die. This case raises a whole spectrum of communication issues and highlights the knowledge and skills students require in order to meet the communication needs of their patients. By considering the case in depth, this chapter will help to equip you with the skills to communicate sensitively and appropriately with patients facing the end of life, and with their families.

CASE STUDY

Mary

Mrs Waters, who likes to be known as Mary, is a 72 year-old married woman living with her husband. She has two adult daughters living some miles away with families of their own. Both Mary and her husband Bill Waters have smoked for most of their lives.

Mary has had chronic obstructive pulmonary disease (COPD) for some years, for which she has regularly taken salbutamol bronchodilator inhalers. She lives with ongoing breathlessness that limits her mobility to around 20 metres, but she manages at home with her husband's help. She enjoys reading romantic novels and in the past was a keen gardener.

Approximately three days ago Mary's breathing worsened considerably, to the point that she struggled to go out at all, and she and Bill went to see her General Practitioner. Mary appeared cyanosed and had a temperature of 38.4 degrees Celsius. She was coughing up thick yellow sputum. Her husband was struggling to care for her at home, and was relieved when the GP advised that she be admitted to their local hospital for treatment of this acute exacerbation of her COPD.

Mary was admitted to an acute medical ward where, despite oxygen therapy, iatripronium inhalers and antibiotic therapy her condition deteriorated further over the next few days. Mary was nursed in a six-bedded open ward so that she could see and be seen by nurses. At this point she required assistance with her personal hygiene each morning, and with walking, which she only did in order to use the toilet. Her speech was impaired by her shortness of breath, and she was becoming extremely tired with the effort of breathing. Bill visited Mary each afternoon, sometimes accompanied by one of their daughters.

Mary was seen by her medical team each morning who advised her of the treatment she was having for this acute infection and exacerbation of her condition. She had had exacerbations of her COPD before and with treatment had made reasonable recoveries. The nurses caring for Mary included Rosie, a second-year student nurse, who had helped her to wash by her bed on a number of shifts. Despite Mary's limited speech she enjoyed Rosie's company and conversation during this task. During a bedside wash one morning, approximately three days into her hospital admission, Mary asked Rosie: 'I'm not getting any better. Am I going to die?'

Rosie struggled to know how to respond.

Reflective questions

Mary and Rosie's situation is a challenging one within health care. Many health care professionals will have been asked this question, perhaps at a time when it has been particularly difficult to answer. It can be challenging both to know what the answer is and how to communicate it sensitively. How might you respond if a patient in Mary's situation asked you this question? You may like to review your answer after reading the whole chapter and consider whether you might respond differently in the future.

Why good communication matters

Experience and common sense suggests that the way we communicate with people, often under difficult circumstances, matters hugely to patients. It shapes relationships and the nature of care. Over the past 20 years clinicians and researchers have explored the significance of communication in health care, particularly end-of-life and cancer care, and good practice is now underpinned by a strong evidence base. Research has emphatically shown that good communication makes a huge difference to patients' experiences of illness and care. This section will consider how communication makes such a difference to patients at the end of their lives, and will also show how health care professionals might use these research findings to shape their everyday practice.

The importance of personal interaction

Richardson (2002) undertook a small study of the interaction between experienced nurses and patients coming to the end of their lives living within the community. Richardson found that patients valued therapeutic interaction with these nurses beyond that necessary simply to complete nursing tasks. The patients valued the sense of being cared for as an individual that the nurses conveyed though their communication. Factors contributing to this therapeutic interaction included the giving of time, being listened to, nurses remembering what patients had said and nurses showing interest and being willing to help. The quality of the relationship positively enhanced patients' feeling of personal well-being. Such interaction is at the heart of nursing patients at the end of their lives. Skills such as listening and showing interest are vital, and can be demonstrated at all levels of health care.

Health care students are well placed to provide personal interaction to patients and should not underestimate the value of doing so. Possible ways of showing interest in patients include asking about their working lives, hobbies and families, picking up a photo from a locker and asking about it, listening attentively to stories and responses and just being pleasant and approachable. It may be appropriate to tell patients a little about yourself, particularly if they ask and show interest, but be aware that this can become burdensome for patients who are likely to be worried about their own situation. Remembering an aspect of a conversation and then asking about it again sometime later can show caring and concern. For example, if a patient says she is worried that her daughter will forget to bring in a clean nightdress, returning later and asking if this happened may feel particularly caring for the patient. Such simple, kind personal interaction may not seem important but, as Richardson's research findings (2002) demonstrate, it conveys a message of being cared about as an individual, which inherently enhances patients' sense of well-being.

Thinking about the case of Mary and Rosie, it would seem likely that over the preceding days Rosie has shown an interest in Mary as a person, and that they have established a personal relationship in which Mary felt able to voice her question.

Dunnice and Slevin (2002) studied the experiences of seven experienced palliative care nurses working in the community. In the context of patients approaching the end of their lives, caring which focuses on 'making people better' by curing their illness is not possible. However, Dunnice and Slevin's research findings (2002) indicate that good communication can help patients *feel better* at the end of their lives simply by sharing their predicament. One of their findings is the significance of 'simply listening' and 'being with' patients, and the potential of these techniques to mitigate isolation and a sense of helplessness. This emphasises the importance of listening attentively, and giving patients time and consideration. Key ways of demonstrating attentive listening include positive non-verbal techniques such as positioning yourself at a similar level to the patient and looking comfortable, preferably seated, to indicate that you plan to listen for a period of time. It is important to maintain eye contact. Nodding your head and giving minimal verbal responses such as 'I see' or 'yes' or 'umm' can let patients know you are listening. Body posture and facial expression are also important. Leaning forward slightly and being upright and alert are all helpful techniques to demonstrate listening.

The case of Mary and Rosie illustrates the importance of communication that takes place alongside common nursing tasks. It is not uncommon for patients to seize the opportunity of a nurse engaged in a practical caring task to raise important concerns. Nurses can demonstrate to patients that they are listening attentively while also undertaking a task by repeating what they have been saying, perhaps by paraphrasing or reflecting. Examples of these techniques are given below.

Reflecting

Reflecting means simply repeating what you have heard:

> *Mary*: Am I going to die, Rosie?
>
> *Rosie*: You are asking me are you going to die?

Paraphrasing

Paraphrasing is similar but this time the response is put into different words:

Mary: Am I going to die, Rosie?

Rosie: You are asking whether you are coming to the end of your life?

Reflecting and paraphrasing what you have heard shows that you have been listening very carefully to the patient and may give them the confidence to say a little more.

Identifying patients' concerns

Research has focused on the importance of communication in identifying patients' concerns accurately to enable patients' needs to be met. Although the importance of communication in assessment is known in the literature, research shows good communication is not always practised sufficiently well to enable thorough assessment. Heaven and Maguire's seminal study of patients in hospices (1997) found that, sadly, the nurses lacked the ability to accurately assess patients' emotional, psychosocial and spiritual concerns. More recently, a study by Farrell et al. (2005) undertaken in a hospital setting found that women undergoing chemotherapy had significant concerns that were not identified by the nurses caring for them; rather, these nurses focused on physical symptoms and treatment-related concerns above psychosocial issues.

Farrell et al. (2005) and Heaven and Maguire's (1997) studies raise some challenging issues for nurses and other health care professionals. They suggest a need to improve communication skills, to expand their assessment beyond the physical and practical, and to encompass a patient's emotional, psychosocial and spiritual concerns. Important practical communication skills that encourage or facilitate patients and families to disclose their concerns in these areas include the following.

Selectively summarising

This means picking up on a particular aspect of what a patient has said to encourage them to say more about it. In the example below, Rosie acknowledges the physical problems Mary has and then focuses on the psychosocial issue raised using Mary's own word: *worried*.

Mary: Oh Rosie it all feels so difficult. I can hardly breathe now and I am really worried. My chest hurts most of the time.

Rosie: You have some problems with your lungs and you're really worried. What is worrying you in particular Mary?

Picking up cues

Often patients wait until they are asked before they disclose their concerns. They may give small hints and try to gauge whether a professional is interested enough to ask. Mostly this is a subconscious process rather than a thought-out strategy. Hints or cues may come in a number of ways. These may include words or phrases that are repeated or particularly emphasised, either by tone of voice or expression, or because they are graphic descriptions. Some may swear in order to emphasise a word or phrase.

Reflective questions

What cues can you find in the following dialogue between Sara, a hospital dietician, and Dave, a 42 year-old man with squamous cell carcinoma of his tonsil receiving radical radiotherapy?

Sara: How are you managing food Dave?

Dave: Well, I'm doing alright I guess, compared to others in here. Can't complain. I mash everything up with my fork so it's nice and mushy and then put it on a spoon to eat. I wouldn't want my kids to see me. Looks like pigs' swill, mind, but it goes down OK. Tastes like pigs' swill too come to think of it.

[Pause, in which Dave looks away, followed by a more upbeat tone.]

I'm holding my own though compared to the others you see. Some of them are walking skeletons. But I'm doing OK, yeah OK.

Dave may be saying he is managing but he has dropped a number of cues that he is not. Describing his food as 'pigs' swill' twice suggests he is distressed by its appearance and taste. The reflective pause may also be a cue that Dave has more to say about this.

Sara could ignore these cues and respond with a physically and practically focused question such as: '*How much have you managed to eat this morning?*' However, if Sara wishes to explore Dave's psychological needs, picking up and reflecting the cue is likely to be more effective: '*The food tastes like pigs' swill?*'

Educated guesses

Making educated guesses can be very helpful in assessing psychological needs. As you read Dave and Sara's dialogue above, you may have found yourself developing ideas of what could be troubling Dave. For example, it may be that in using comparisons with patients around him, he is trying hard to disassociate from them as he is frightened of becoming as sick as they are. Alternatively, he may be distressed by the manner in which he now has to eat, and is anxious about having family meals in the future. Such ideas are only guesses, but, if presented tentatively so that patients can refute them if needs be, educated guesses can help health care professionals and patients clarify their concerns. To offer an educated guess Sara could say something like:

Sara: Dave, listening to you I am wondering if seeing such poorly people in here makes you worry about your own future.

Or:

I may be wrong, but I imagine family meals may be a real worry for you when you go home.

Action point

This section has explored the significance of good communication and the techniques that facilitate it. Consider which, if any, you tend to use, perhaps inadvertently. Next time you are in practice, notice when more experienced professionals use them. Finally, try them out for yourself!

Poor communication

Given the significance of good communication, it is unsurprising that research shows that poor communication is detrimental to patient care. Poor communication is that in which meaningful exchange has not effectively taken place; rather, it has been inappropriately blocked by the health care professional, leaving the patient and relative confused, unheard or misinformed. Thorne, Bults and Baile (2005) reviewed the research literature which addressed the impact of poor communication in cancer care and found that it has a significant negative impact on psychosocial experience, symptom management, treatment decision and quality of life. In addition, a study by Thorne et al. (2004) into communication with patients living with multiple sclerosis shows the potential of poor communication to undermine patients' ability to manage their own care and needs. Indeed, poor communication is one of the main causes of patients' complaints overall (Healthcare Commission 2008). Poor communication, or communication that is blocked by health professionals, is explored in more detail in the next section.

Blocking and facilitating communication strategies

The work of Thorne et al. (2004) has shown the impact on patients when health care professionals block patients from expressing their concerns and communicating their worries. Professionals may be unaware that they are communicating in ways that block patients. Blocking communication can easily become an inadvertent habit, so becoming aware of personal blocking strategies is vital for self-awareness and the development of more effective communication. Common blocking strategies are shown below, together with contrasting facilitative strategies which aim to enable patients to disclose their concerns.

Normalising

Normalising is suggesting something is insignificant because it is common. Normalising blocks communication about something that is in fact hugely significant to the patient.

> *Mary*: I feel really tired and wiped out all the time.

> *Rosie*: Oh everyone feels like that in the winter.

Of course Rosie may be right but this statement is unlikely to encourage Mary to talk further about the fact that the tiredness she is feeling is likely to be due to her illness. A more helpful response that encourages the patient to discuss her worries might be:

> *Rosie*: I've noticed how tired you seem. How long has this been the case?

Giving reassurance prematurely (before the patient has disclosed their full concern):

> *Mary*: My husband has not come to visit me again today.

> *Rosie*: I am sure he will come in this evening.

Once again Rosie has closed the subject, possibly making it very difficult for Mary to say more. An alternative might be:

> *Rosie*: He's not visited?

> *Mary*: It was all getting too much for him at home. I don't know if he will want me back there.

Premature advice

> *Mary*: I don't think I can manage these tablets.

> *Rosie*: Just take your time, try taking the bigger ones first and washing them down with this water.

In this situation Mary is left with little option but to drink the water. An alternative reply which explores Mary's concerns more thoroughly might be:

> *Rosie*: What problems are you having, Mary?

> *Mary*: The antibiotics are making me feel sick.

From this second piece of dialogue we can see that Rosie's initial advice was premature and unhelpful. By exploring Mary's concerns further, Rosie can offer much more appropriate care.

False reassurance

Mary: I think I may be dying.

Rosie: Don't talk like that Mary. You will be OK.

Rosie has stopped Mary from talking about her impending death with reassurance that may not be true. Later, the chapter will explore how such difficult questions might be answered more openly.

Passing the buck

The example below gives a possible response to Mary's disclosure of some of her concerns:

Mary: I have not slept a wink all night worrying about money.

Rosie: I will refer you to the social worker for benefits advice.

In this case, rather than exploring Mary's concerns at all, Rosie 'passes the buck' to the social worker, promptly closing the subject and blocking any further discussion. An alternative response that explores the concern further could be:

Rosie: What is it that is bothering you, Mary?

Mary: I think I should make a will.

From this exploration, we can see that referral to a social worker for benefits advice was in fact inappropriate.

Jollying along

Rosie [approaching Mary who looks sad]: Come on Mary, it's a lovely sunny day out today...

Although such a positive comment may be well meant, it stops Mary from explaining why she feels sad.

Reflective questions

Consider the impact of blocking techniques on patients like Mary. Take the following piece of dialogue:

> *Mary*: I think I may be dying.

> *Rosie*: Don't talk like that, Mary, you will be OK.

How do you imagine Mary might feel following Rosie's response?

Thinking of Rosie and Mary, consider the following possible responses Rosie might give to Mary's question of 'Am I going to die?'

> I don't think so.

> What makes you ask that?

> Sorry mmmm....

> Mary I just need to check on Joan next door.

Add any other response that you think you might give if you were in Rosie's shoes. Consider each in turn. Do you think they are likely to block Mary from talking further or support her in disclosing her worries?

Why health care professionals block communication with dying patients and their families

Blocking behaviour by health care professionals is understandable. Caring for patients at the end of their lives can be extremely daunting, particularly if it is new and unfamiliar. This section explores why health care professionals might find care of the dying difficult and shy away from complex conversations with both dying patients and their families.

At the beginning of the twentieth century, death commonly occurred at home in the presence of family members. Those same family members would have cared for the sick person. Generally, people would have had experience of seeing and being involved in the care of the dying, and may therefore have had some understanding of how to respond to the needs of the dying and the bereaved. (The care for dying people over the past century is explored in greater detail in Chapter 1).

By contrast, in contemporary Britain people have far less experience of death. Throughout the country only 18% of people die at home (Department of Health 2008), and while family care is still given, it is likely to be managed by health care professionals. As a result, in general, people now have much less experience of death and dying.

Even those entering the health care professions may have had very little contact with dying or bereaved people.

Communicating with dying patients in any depth can be frightening for a number of reasons. Cooper and Barnett's investigation (2005) of first-year student nurses' anxieties about caring for dying patients found that student nurses are often worried about how to cope with:

- witnessing the physical suffering of dying patients;
- being upset when a patient they had known died;
- saying 'the wrong thing';
- making patients feel worse than they already do;
- unexpected death; and
- carrying out last offices.

Sometimes the fear is based more in professional activity and the demands of the health care environment than in their personal reaction. Nurses may worry about conversations taking up too much time, that they may be seen as 'doing nothing' or that as students they are 'not allowed' to discuss sensitive issues. Clarke and Ross's (2006) study exploring the factors influencing nurses' (including student nurses) communication, found that the culture of the working environment significantly influences the way nurses communicate. When nurses feel torn between the needs of different patients or conflicting priorities (such as whether to spend half an hour attending a multidisciplinary meeting or completing a patient audit form), they may feel unable to prioritise time to listen to dying patients.

The consequence of such understandable anxieties and conflicts in caring for those who are dying may be that professionals tend to distance themselves from the situation in some way. Essentially this may be to protect themselves against the emotional risks of engaging with patients at a deeper level, such as being presented with suffering or feeling sad about the death of someone they have personally cared for. Common distancing strategies identified in student nurses include trying to 'detach' or 'switch off' their personal feelings, being busy or talking about 'happy subjects' (Cooper and Barnett 2005). Registered staff have similar concerns and responses to students, though this may be less apparent. Seminal research by Susie Wilkinson (1991), in which she studied the communication of 54 registered nurses working with cancer patients, found overall that nurses gave very poor or no coverage at all to psychosocial aspects of care. While there was wide variation between individual nurses, overall blocking rather than facilitative communication dominated, particularly in the assessment of patients whose cancer had recurred. This discouraged patients from telling the nurses of their concerns.

While blocking techniques are generally unhelpful, they may be appropriate in some circumstances. It may well be inadvisable to encourage patient disclosure of concerns and worries at a particular time, for example when in the middle of a drug round or just before you have an important appointment. In this situation it is important to acknowledge the circumstances so that the patient is aware that the opportunity will be available in the future. An example of this is given below:

> *Mary*: I feel absolutely exhausted today. I don't understand why, Rosie.

> *Rosie*: I can see you are, Mary. I would like to talk about this with you. When I have finished the drug round I will come back.

Rosie has purposefully blocked Mary but has indicated that she will be available in the future.

Patients, and indeed most people, also use blocking techniques when they do not wish to discuss something. Faced with a looming deadline to hand in an assignment, it is tempting to spend precious time on other matters (often cleaning out kitchen cupboards in my experience!). Similarly, faced with an overwhelming worry, such as whether or not death is imminent, some patients will want to talk about anything else to avoid discussing their concern. It is important to recognise and respect their wishes and behaviour. Avoidance can be a positive way of living with overwhelming worry. The role of the health professional is simply to *offer* patients the opportunity to disclose their concerns and worries, and many will choose not to take it up. Continue to offer that opportunity so that if patients choose, they can take it up when they are ready.

In the example below, Rosie respects Mary's block of the opportunity to discuss her worries at that time, but makes it clear the opportunity remains.

> *Rosie*: Mary, you don't seem quite yourself today. Is there anything on your mind?

> *Mary*: Oh not really, How was your night out yesterday?

> *Rosie* [after talking a little about the night out, then, perhaps later, saying]: Do ask if you have any questions about anything, Mary.

Blocking techniques will close down communication. While their use is often inadvertent and develops for very understandable reasons, they can leave patients feeling isolated, unable to share what is on their minds. However, used purposefully they can protect both practitioners and patients from unwanted discussions.

Action point

Awareness of your own use of blocking techniques, and the development of skills to use them only when they are helpful, is key to improving good communication. Consider if and how you block communication.

Who should respond to difficult questions?

Reflective question

If you were in Rosie's shoes, consider whether you could be the right person to answer Mary's question? If not, how might you respond to Mary?

Students commonly worry that they are 'not allowed' to answer patients' difficult questions. It may be that they lack the information or knowledge to answer the question correctly or that they lack the skill to answer it sensitively. Sometimes students feel they lack the authority to respond to significant questions. Clearly it is important that students recognise the limitations of their current knowledge and skills, and seek guidance and support when appropriate. In doing so, it is important to let the patient know that, while support is required to give an answer, the question is important and will be taken seriously. A way of showing this is given below:

Mary: Am I going to die?

Rosie: Mary, that is a difficult question and to be honest I need some help to answer it. What has made you wonder about that?

Mary: Well, I feel absolutely rotten. Last time the tablets brought me round in a few days but this time they aren't doing much. No one has said anything about changing them but I can't go on like this.

Rosie: Is there anything else that is worrying you, Mary?

Mary: I am really worried about Bill, you know; how he will cope and that.

Rosie: You've got a lot on your mind – the treatment is not helping and you're worried about what will happen to Bill in the future. I would like to tell Nick, the staff nurse, about this and then come back to you. Would that be OK with you?

In a situation like the one described above, Rosie has acknowledged Mary's concerns and offered a strategy to address them. It is important that students remain involved in responding to patients' concerns. Rosie could choose to come back to Mary with Nick and observe him in responding to Mary's concerns. Alternatively, she could talk the situation through with Nick, and then respond to Mary directly, either with or without Nick present. Such conversations can be rich sources of learning particularly when reflected on in depth, perhaps using a structured model of reflection such as those described by Gibbs (1988) or Johns (2004). These models enable you to consider what happened in a conversation in some detail, and allow you to think about what, if anything, you may choose to do differently in future. The structure of Gibbs' (1988) model is given in Figure 3.1.

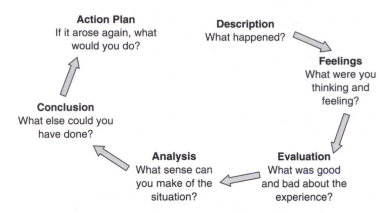

Figure 3.1   Gibbs' reflective cycle (1988)

Many practical communication skills may be learnt by making a mental note of the phrases and techniques used by more experienced professionals. This will build a repertoire that can be drawn upon in future. Some of these phrases can be recalled verbatim; others can be put into similar words that come more intuitively. Different communication styles can be equally effective as long as the key principles are observed.

Action point

When you are in practice, build your own 'tool box' of phrases you find helpful and are comfortable using. If, on reflection, you think 'I wish I had said that!', metaphorically put it in your 'tool box' for another time. If you notice a phrase that someone else uses effectively, make it your own. If you hear something you think did not work well, reflect on how you might phrase it more effectively.

Recognising that someone is approaching the end of his or her life can be very difficult. Full consideration of the physical signs is given in Chapter 8. However, the end of someone's natural life cannot be accurately predicted. Living with an uncertainty about the future is often very difficult both for patients and for their families. This is particularly so in a contemporary culture which values reliability and clarity. Responding to difficult questions relating to the end of life involves breaking bad news, and is therefore challenging. The next section will focus on how this might best be achieved.

Breaking bad news sensitively

There is a significant body of literature which has specifically considered best practice when breaking bad news to patients. A classic definition of bad news is given by

Buckman (1992: 15) as 'any news that drastically and negatively alters a patient's view of his or her future'. It is information that changes a person's view of themselves, his or her current and future situation, and/or relationships in a profoundly unwelcome or negative way. As such, breaking bad news is difficult. It is rarely experienced as a single event but is an ongoing process of communication, often punctuated by significant conversations, by which patients become informed of and internalise the news (Salander 2002). It is a process which involves the whole multidisciplinary care team, albeit with differing contributions. Nurses, for example, are likely to be involved in monitoring patients' awareness of their condition, managing the consequences of bad news for patients and addressing their subsequent psychological needs. If we look at Mary's case, clearly Mary is expecting bad news. Rosie is in a position to identify and manage her concerns, though she may not have sufficient knowledge and skill to give the bad news herself.

A number of guidelines of good practice have been devised which provide frameworks for breaking bad news, such as advancing life-threatening illness, sensitively (Buckman 1992; Kaye 1996; Baile et al. 2000). While the evidence base supporting their use is limited, they provide helpful reminders of important points. Peter Kaye's 10-step model of breaking bad news is given below, together with advice for how it might be followed and some potential pitfalls to be avoided.

1. Preparation

Being well prepared to break bad news is vital. Before doing so:

- make sure you know all the facts;
- prepare the environment by finding out who the patient wants to be present;
- go somewhere private;
- be on the same physical level as the patient/relatives.

When relating this to Mary and Rosie's case, it may be that Rosie genuinely does not know the answer to Mary's question and needs to find out before she can answer it.

2. What does the patient want to know?

Patients and relatives may ask health professionals difficult questions about life expectancy or health in a number of ways. Sometimes they ask '*Am I going to die?*' or '*Am I dying?*' Others might ask '*How long have I got to live?*' or something more specific, such as: '*Will I see Christmas?*' Patients and relatives ask these questions for a number of reasons. Patients may want to plan for their limited future or they may be hoping that their fears are unfounded. Relatives may be asking for information so that they can plan leave from work or a holiday away. It is vital to clarify what specifically is being asked and for what purpose. Ask for a narrative to find out the patient's current understanding and what he or she is currently asking. Some ways of asking this include: 'How did it all start?' or 'What have the doctors told you so far?' Rosie might ask Mary: 'What makes you ask me that now, Mary?'

3. Is more information wanted?

Patients and relatives raising difficult questions about the end of life may simply be voicing a thought aloud without ever wanting it to be answered. Therefore it is important to offer further information rather than give what is not wanted.

For example: 'Would you like me to explain a bit more? Or would you like to know the answer to that question now?'

4. Give a warning shot

It may be helpful to give some warning of bad news. For example: 'I am afraid things are not as good as we hoped.'

5. Allow denial

If patients indicate that they do not want more information or to continue with the conversation, respect this.

6. Explain (if requested)

Give the information clearly and step by step. Give the chance to stop you if they wish to voice concerns or ask questions. If this happens, check whether they want more information before continuing. Take a tentative approach, explaining that it is impossible to accurately predict future health or death. For example, Rosie might respond to Mary:

> *Rosie*: As you know, the tablets you had last year worked very well, but disappointingly this time they have not had much effect. The test we have done on your lungs shows that your illness has worsened since then. ... We can't be sure how things will go now. It may be that your health will improve, but it is also possible that it will get worse, I am afraid. If that happens, yes, you could die from this infection.

Avoid euphemisms for death that may confuse patents and relatives such as: 'We could lose you.'

Do include words that express your sadness about the news, such as 'I am sorry. We are disappointed.'

7. Listen to concerns

Listen carefully if patients raise worries and concerns about this news. You may ask if they have any questions. Avoid false and premature reassurance of any concern which might block communication.

8. Encourage ventilation of feelings

Take time to listen sensitively to patients' feelings following bad news. Patients and relatives react in many different ways. Many will be sad, perhaps tearful; others may be relieved to have shared and discussed their fears. For some, the news will be a shock; for others a confirmation of what they already know. It is possible that what health care professionals expect to be devastating can be welcome to a patient. Some patients and/or relatives become angry and may verbalise this strongly and unpleasantly. Try to remember that usually such anger is not personal, but is a result of the sad situation that they face.

It is tempting to try to make things better at this stage by normalising or being optimistic. Phrases such as: *'Don't worry, I'm sure everything will turn out OK'* are not helpful. Remember it is not possible to make bad news into good news.

Some nurses find themselves getting upset together with patients and relatives facing sad news. When this is genuine compassion it is usually valued by families. However, it is important that the focus of care remains firmly with the patient and family rather that the nurse. If you find yourself overwhelmed by sadness, seek support from your mentor and colleagues rather than from patients and their families!

Physically touching patients, perhaps on the hand or embracing, can also show compassion and care. However, on the other hand, it can be uncomfortable. If you wish to touch in this way, first consider if this is likely to be helpful and then approach it tentatively, perhaps by placing your hand near or saying: *'Would it be OK to give you a hug?'*

9. Summary and plan

Summarise any concerns and offer a plan for how to proceed. To achieve this, Rosie might say to Mary:

> Rosie: I can see how worried you are that the antibiotics are not working this time, and that you are getting worse rather than better. I will make sure the doctors know this so they can review your treatment.

10. Offer availability

Patients may need to discuss the news further. They are likely to struggle to remember everything and may have questions later on. Make sure they know whom to contact with questions and how to do so. This might be as simple as saying '*I will call back in half an hour to see if there is anything else you would like to ask.*'

Reflective question

Peter Kaye's guidelines can be applied widely. Imagine you are a newly-qualified staff nurse working on a surgical ward. One of your patients, Edward, is eagerly planning to go home tomorrow but crucially needs a hoist to be delivered to his home. Unfortunately its delivery has been delayed until after the weekend. Using Kaye's guidance to break this bad news to Edward, what might you say to him at each stage?

Action point

This chapter has given examples of responses to difficult communication issues. You may find some phrases here that you are comfortable with saying yourself, but others that are not your style. Remember that there are usually a number of ways to convey the same thing. Watch more experienced practitioners at work and build a collection of phrases that you consider effective and feel comfortable using. It is also possible to learn from phrases that you feel did not help communication. Clearly these are to be avoided!

Action point

Listening is usually far more effective than talking. Attentive listening can convey caring and concern. If you find yourself stuck for words, simply say genuinely: 'I just don't know what to say to you' or 'I just don't know what I can say that might help you right now'.

Sources of support for students

Always talk to your mentor or personal tutor if you are finding caring for dying patients emotionally difficult. Alternatively, most universities offer confidential counselling services and advice lines. There is more information about sources of support in Chapter 12.

Returning to Mary's case

Rosie successfully explores Mary's question and discovers that Mary is simply voicing her fear that she is not getting any better, and that she is not expecting Rosie to answer the question directly. Mary appreciated being able to share her fears with Rosie.

Action point

Review any notes you have made on how you might have responded to Mary's question. Would you change your response, and if so, what in particular has changed your approach?

Summary

The key points to remember when faced with difficult questions are:

- Communication is a key determinant of quality care.
- Communicating with dying patients is challenging for all professionals and often daunting for students.
- Using a model of breaking bad news can help to answer difficult questions.
- As a student, it may be better to seek help if faced with a difficult question from a patient, but be careful to acknowledge the importance of the question and ensure that it is answered.

Further reading

Dunphy, J. (2011) *Communication in Palliative Care: Clear Practical Advice, Based on a Series of Real Case Studies*. Oxford: Radcliffe Publishing.
Written by an experienced clinical nurse specialist in palliative care, Dunphy shares her experience in communicating with patients at the end of life through stories full of tips and sensible advice. This book is readable and engaging.

Webb, L. (2011) *Nursing: Communication Skills in Practice*. Oxford: Oxford University Press.
This book is written specifically for student nurses. It aims to relate communication theory to practice across a range of clinical fields. Although it is not specifically focused on communication in end-of-life care, it provides up-to-date and valuable reading required within the Nursing and Midwifery Council Competency Framework (2010).

Ghaye, A. and Lillyman, S. (2011) *When Caring Is Not Enough: Examples of Reflection in Practice*. London: Quay Books

This book is recommended for learning about reflection and its usefulness in helping health care professionals make sense of and learn from challenging situations.

National End of Life Care Programme (2011) *Finding the Words* [online]. Available at: www.endoflifecareforadults.nhs.uk/publications/finding-the-words [accessed 28 April 2012]. This workbook and DVD has been devised by the National End of Life Care Programme for people with a life-limiting illness and for bereaved people. It uses the real experiences of patients and carers to support health and social professionals develop communication skills.

References

Baile, W., Buckman, R., Lenzi, R., Gobler, G., Beale, E.A. and Kudelka, A.P. (2000) 'Spikes: a six-step protocol for delivering bad news: application to the patient suffering from cancer', *Oncologist*, 5(4): 302–11.

Buckman, R. (1992) *How to Break Bad News: A Guide for Healthcare Professionals*. Baltimore, MD: Johns Hopkins University Press.

Clarke, A. and Ross, H. (2006) 'Influences on nurses' communications with older people at the end of life: perceptions and experiences of nurses working in palliative care and general medicine', *International Journal of Older People Nursing*, 1: 34–43.

Cooper, J. and Barnett, M. (2005) 'Aspects of caring for dying patients which cause anxiety to first-year student nurses', *International Journal of Palliative Nursing*, 11(8): 423–30.

Department of Health (2008) *End of Life Care Strategy*. London: DH.

Dunnice, U. and Slevin, E. (2002) 'Giving voice to the less articulated knowledge of palliative nursing: an interpretive study', *International Journal of Palliative Nursing*, 8(1): 13–20.

Farrell, C., Heaven, C., Beaver, K. and Maguire, P. (2005) 'Identifying the concerns of women undergoing chemotherapy', *Patient Education and Counselling*, 56: 72–7.

Gibbs, G. (1988) *Learning by Doing: A Guide to Teaching and Learning Methods*. Oxford: Further Education Unit, Oxford Polytechnic.

Healthcare Commission (2008) *Spotlight on Complaints*. London: Commission for Healthcare Audit and Inspection.

Heaven, C. and Maguire, P. (1997) 'Disclosure of concerns by hospice patients and their identification by nurses', *Palliative Medicine*, 11(4): 283–90.

Johns, C. (2004) *Becoming a Reflective Practitioner* (2nd edn). Oxford: Blackwell.

Kaye, P. (1996) *Breaking Bad News: A 10-Step Approach*. Northampton: EPL Publications.

Richardson, J. (2002) 'Health promotion in palliative care: the patients' perception of therapeutic interaction with the palliative nurse in the primary care setting', *Journal of Advanced Nursing*, 40(4): 432–40.

Salander, P. (2002) 'Bad news from the patient's perspective: an analysis of the written narratives of newly-diagnosed cancer patients', *Social Science in Medicine*, 55(5): 721–32.

Thorne, S., Bults, B. and Baile, W. (2005) 'Is there a cost to poor communication? A critical review of the literature', *Psychooncology*, 14(10): 875–84.

Thorne, S., Con, A., McGinness, L., McPherson, G. and Harries, S. (2004) 'Healthcare communication issues in multiple sclerosis: an interpretive description', *Qualitative Health Research*, 14(1): 5–22.

Wilkinson, S. (1991) 'Factors which influence how nurses communicate with cancer patients', *Journal of Advanced Nursing*, 16: 677–88.

CHAPTER 4

Making difficult decisions using ethical and legal frameworks

Annie Pettifer

This chapter will explore:

- The key ethical principles
- The doctrine of double effect
- Key legal aspects of decision-making at the end of life
- How a patient's ability to make a decision is assessed
- How decisions are made regarding care of people who cannot express their own wishes
- How people may influence decisions that may be made about them if they lose capacity in the future
- The role of the health care student in end-of-life care decision-making

Introduction

Patients reaching the end of their lives, their relatives and professional carers often face difficult decisions about how patients spend the remaining time they have to live, and how they are cared for. Currently, health care policy in the United

Kingdom places great emphasis on providing people with choices about their care (Department of Health 2008). Nurses are often in the position of assisting people to make decisions about these choices. The following case study raises a range of important issues of difficult decision-making when someone is facing the end of their life. While the case focuses on an older woman with diagnosed dementia, the issues it raises can relate to patients in a variety of situations as well as to their families and health care practitioners. By exploring these vital issues in depth, this chapter will equip you to deliver your role in supporting and assisting patients, families and practitioners with difficult decisions in these situations.

CASE STUDY

Edith

Mrs Tuckman, who likes to be known as Edith, is an 84 year-old woman living with multi-infarct dementia and progressive heart failure. Edith has been married and has raised three sons who are now living in different parts of the country, two with families of their own. Edith has suffered with increasing multi-infarct dementia for the last six years. Initially she was cared for at home by her husband, but when he died suddenly two years ago Edith moved into a nursing care home. At first, Edith was able to meet some of her own care needs, as long as she was prompted by staff. She enjoyed a good sing at the piano and visits from her sons. However, over time Edith's dementia worsened. During the last six months, Edith has had repeated infections, usually precipitating admission to the local hospital. With antibiotic therapy, Edith has recovered, but her quality of life has slowly diminished and she does not seem to enjoy music anymore.

Charlotte, a third-year student nurse, is halfway through an eight-week placement at the nursing home in which Edith resides. She has cared for Edith over the last couple of weeks and had come to know her a little. One morning Charlotte went to help Edith eat her breakfast and found her hot and sweaty. Edith was coughing quite a bit but in-between seemed drowsy and lethargic. Charlotte noticed green phlegm in the tissue Edith was clutching. Alerting the staff nurse Janet to this, they found Edith's temperature to be 38.2 degrees Celsius and her pulse 94 beats per minute. They gave her some water and 1g of paracetamol. Janet phoned Edith's General Practitioner (GP) and requested a visit later that day. At Janet's request, Charlotte telephoned Barry, Edith's nearest son, to let him know that Edith was not well and that the GP would visit later in the day. During this conversation Barry said how sad it was to see Edith's health deteriorating, and that she seemed to get less and less pleasure from living. He hoped that Dr Cooper would not send her to hospital or put her through any more unpleasant treatments. Last time she took antibiotics she found them very difficult to swallow and they gave her diarrhoea, although her chest infection had abated. He mentioned that his sister, Sarah, had 'legal responsibility' and he would ask her what she thought.

Later Edith's temperature decreased and she seemed a little brighter, although her cough was still troublesome and productive. Dr Cooper, Edith's GP, arrived and indeed diagnosed that Edith had a chest infection and was in need of antibiotics. Charlotte told him of Barry's thoughts about treatment and hospitalisation. She wondered what Dr Cooper would do.

In situations such as this it can be difficult to discern the right course of action. There are key ethical principles and legal requirements in place to assist with decision-making, and these will be discussed in this chapter.

The key ethical principles

Beauchamp and Childress (2001) describe four ethical principles of beneficence, non-maleficence, autonomy and justice that provide a helpful and widely-established framework for considering ethical dilemmas. Principles are notions or high standards that carry authority and respect. They are helpful and usually guide practice, but it is important to remember that they may be legitimately overridden in some circumstances. Ethical decisions are, by their nature, difficult to make, and sometimes when each of the four principles is applied, they conflict in some way. For example, a decision that is beneficent for a patient may not necessarily be beneficent for their relative.

Beneficence and non-maleficence

The older two of the four principles are beneficence and non-maleficence. Beneficence can be defined as 'the duty to do good for others'; non-maleficence is rather different and can be defined as 'the duty to do no harm'.

Originally, beneficence was meant in the sense of being a Good Samaritan or offering a noble service. In health care it has come to mean doing what is good for patients. Obviously people, whether health care professionals or family members, may vary in their view of what is good for a patient. Their views are likely to be shaped by a whole range of factors, including their values, hopes and beliefs. There may be disagreement between different individuals or groups of people about what is good for a patient and this may make decision-making very difficult.

There is an obvious difficulty in applying beneficence in Edith's case. Barry, her son, considers that 'doing good' for Edith means not giving her antibiotics and that nature should take its course. The GP, however, may feel that giving antibiotics is the most beneficent action. When there is conflict in a decision-making process, it is important to remember that each person in the patient's team is trying to decide what is best for the patient based on their values and, in the case of health care professionals, their professional standards and training. In order for multidisciplinary teamworking to be effective, everyone's views need to be respectfully considered as part of the decision-making process. In this way patient care is enriched by a number of perspectives (Pettifer et al. 2007).

Reflective questions

In turn, consider the motivation and thinking behind the decisions reached by:

1　Barry
2　Dr Cooper

Reflect on each of these perspectives. Which do you consider to be the 'right thing' for Edith?

What is the value of considering both of these points of view together?

Action point

Be sensitive to your colleagues in ethical decision-making. When the views of your colleagues are different from your own, they are likely simply to have a different view of what is in the patient's best interest.

Interestingly, non-maleficence was originally meant in the sense of not practising outside the scope of one's ability, but has come to be understood much more literally as not doing anything to a patient that may hurt or harm them. Florence Nightingale was clearly a protagonist of non-maleficence, because in the 1860s hospitals were places very likely to harm patients, as she herself recognised:

> It may seem a strange principle to enunciate as the very first requirement in a hospital is that it should do the sick no harm. It is quite necessary, nevertheless, to lay down such a principle, because the actual mortality in hospitals, especially those of large crowded cities, is very much higher than any calculation founded on the mortality of the same class of diseases among patients treated out of hospital would lead us to expect. (Nightingale 1863: 1)

Sadly, unintentionally harming patients is still a real possibility today. A patient may be admitted to hospital with the best intentions of improving their health only to acquire an infection from the hospital environment which debilitates them further. Often the possibility of harm is foreseeable and needs to be carefully weighed against the potential for benefit. For example, cytoxic chemotherapy may be very effective against malignant cells but will also damage healthy tissue, causing unpleasant and harmful side-effects. If the principle of non-maleficence is applied to Edith's case, we might reasonably argue that antibiotics may harm her by causing diarrhoea, and therefore should not be given. However, they may also improve her condition by treating the infection. Clearly, the balance of these two effects has to be carefully weighed.

Autonomy

Beneficence and non-maleficence were for a long time the dominant principles of western health care. Essentially they supported health care professionals' authority to make decisions that, in their judgement, based on their expert knowledge and experience, were good for their patients. This approach is strongly paternalistic, suggesting that it is reasonable for one person with authority to make important decisions about another as long as they are caring for them, much as a parent might for their child. However, following the Second World War, attitudes to health care began to change, reflecting an increase in expectations across society as a whole. For example, in 1960 it became clear that in some cases, consent had not been obtained for dangerous research, and as a consequence research ethics committees were formed to protect the rights of individuals (Randall and Downie 2001). Thus the principle of autonomy, or *self*-rule, began to hold more authority. Autonomy in a health care context is the principle of people making their own decisions based on their own values and beliefs. These decisions may or may not differ from those of health professionals, but the key aspect is that they are made by the individual for and about themselves. When autonomy is prized above beneficence, the role of health care professionals becomes one of offering relevant information and choice; their role is to enable a decision, rather than making the decision themselves. The increasing influence of the principle of autonomy can be seen across much of contemporary government policy in the United Kingdom. For example, in the field of education, parents are offered a choice of schools, and information is published to support parents in making their choice. Autonomy has been particularly supported within the nursing profession, with nurses keen to position themselves as advocates, supporting patients in making decisions about their own health care.

The principle of autonomy is not without its pitfalls. Thoresen (2003) argues that expecting very sick patients (who are likely to be exhausted) to weigh information and make difficult decisions related to their well-being simply adds to their already considerable burden. Some patients, of whom Edith is one, are simply unable to assess the information given to them and make decisions due to the effects of the disease they have. Other patients may simply not wish to consider, make and then live with difficult choices and would prefer others to do this on their behalf. In addition, any decision made by upholding the principle of one person's autonomy may challenge another's autonomy. For example, perhaps a woman decides she wishes to be cared for and die at home, but her husband and only potential carer in the house does not wish to care for her there. While it may be possible to uphold her decision without his support, it is likely that he will be asked to care for her at some time, thus compromising his own wishes.

Autonomy tends to be dominant in contemporary western society where individualism is valued. Others may value a much more collective approach in which the whole family's wishes take precedence over the individual. For example, in traditional Chinese culture the principle of autonomy has little authority as individuals are considered an integral part of the family. Family members will therefore expect to have a huge influence in any decision involving an individual patient. It is expected that discussing terminal illness is likely to worry a sick individual and, therefore, in a spirit of beneficence, families are likely to see themselves as the appropriate people with whom to discuss illness and want information to be withheld from the individual (Chater and Tsai 2008).

Justice

Beauchamp and Childress' (2001) fourth key ethical principle is that of justice, or fairness. This usually refers to the fair use and distribution of finite and limited resources. In health care it is particularly relevant as the major resource is professional time. This presents a challenge to every health care professional, who must be concerned with decisions about how to allocate their time and expertise fairly. However, there are differing approaches to fair distribution of resources. The principle of utility demands that resources are used to benefit the greatest number to the greatest extent. The principle of equity demands that the resource is evenly spread. Sometimes a tension between the two arises. For example, following the principle of utility, it might be desirable to base a nurse who is a specialist in end-of-life care within a nursing home where there is a concentration of patients who may require such expertise. However, this may not follow the principle of equity as those who live outside the nursing home may have less access to such specialist care. The principle of equity demands that the nurse spreads his or her service evenly to all.

The principle of justice plays little part in the decision as to whether or not Edith should have antibiotics as no resource limitations are presented within the case. However, in a situation where only three courses of antibiotic were available and Edith was one of ten patients who might benefit from them, the decision would be difficult. On one hand, equity demands those antibiotics should be distributed evenly across all ten patients. This may be fair but if the dose is insufficient, it will have a limited effect on those ten. Utility demands that the antibiotics are given to only three patients who would benefit the most, while the other seven would not recieve antibiotics at all. This involves a difficult decision concerning which three should be treated.

Reflective question

Imagine that you are, like Charlotte, nursing Edith for the shift. You are also required to care for other patients in the nursing home with a range of nursing needs. Like many nurses, you will need to consider how best to use your time to care for all these patients.

Edith is frightened of being alone in case she chokes on the phlegm from her chest infection, and she asks you to sit with her. Another patient in your care, Hannah, regularly likes a morning bath at this time.

Applying the ethical principles of, first, equity and then utility, consider how you might allocate the key resource of your time. Is your decision different depending on which principle is followed? If so, which principle are you more comfortable with and why?

The doctrine of double effect

In addition to the four key ethical principles relevant to end-of-life care, we also need to consider the 'doctrine of double effect'. This doctrine upholds a decision where the intention when it was made was positive, even if, sadly, the outcome of the decision was not. For the doctrine of double effect to hold, a decision must be made in the belief that the positive effects of the decision made will outweigh any potential negative effects it causes. The negative effects may be foreseen but not intended, and should not outweigh the positive effects. The negative effect cannot itself be the intention (Thorns 1998). To continue the earlier example of chemotherapy, the intention of giving cytotoxic chemotherapy is to treat cancer. We can foresee that unpleasant side-effects will occur, but they are not intended. Their unpleasantness is usually outweighed by the patient's desire for treatment. In this example, the doctrine of double effect is upheld, and the decision to give cytotoxic chemotherapy is ethical and legal despite its unpleasant side-effects.

In Edith's case, the GP's decision to give antibiotics clearly follows the doctrine of double effect. His intention is to treat her infection and to relieve her suffering, even though the negative effect is that the antibiotics will potentially cause diarrhoea. On balance, however, he feels that treating the underlying infection is a better outcome for Edith than the temporary suffering she will experience from the diarrhoea.

Key legal aspect of decision-making at the end of life

The key ethical principles described above can help explore the clinical dilemma that Charlotte faces. However, as we have seen, they may conflict, and their application can be subjective. For example, one clinician may value a paternalistic approach to decision-making and another may favour an approach based on autonomy. In contrast, Acts of Parliament provide law that is imperative, and is intended to apply regardless of individual clinicians' personal points of view (Griffin and Tengnah 2010). Difficult decisions concerning end of life are governed by legislation and influenced by ethical principles. As the chapter continues, key legal frameworks are described and how legal and ethical decisions about end-of-life care are made in practice will be discussed in detail.

How a patient's ability to make a decision is assessed

As described above, although autonomy is the key ethical principle governing much of western health care at this time, some patients cannot exercise their autonomy and make decisions. This may be because they have either a temporary or permanent impairment which is affecting their ability to do so. For example, they may have an acute infection causing temporary confusion or brain metastases (cancer that has spread to the brain) causing cognitive impairment.

The Mental Capacity Act 2005 (UK Parliament 2005) provides a legally-binding framework, both for assessing a patient's ability to make decisions and also for decision-making processes in circumstances when patients lack this ability. Unlike the key ethical principles which underpin ethical thinking but do not give prescriptive guidance for practice, the Mental Capacity Act is legally binding and health care professionals must adhere to its provisions.

The Mental Capacity Act 2005 requires that all patients must be assumed to have the ability (termed 'capacity') to make their own decisions unless it has been established that they cannot do so. When required, people must be supported as much as is practicable to make decisions, for example, by providing information in Braille or by using particular communication aides or styles (such as taking care to face the patient when talking to him or her). However, if a patient remains unable to make a decision despite all efforts to assist decision-making, it may be that the patient lacks the capacity to make the particular decision and this should be assessed under the terms of the Act.

Under the terms of the Mental Capacity Act 2005, a person is lacking in capacity if:

- they have an impairment or disturbance (e.g. a disability, condition or trauma) that affects the way their mind or brain works, and
- the impairment or disturbance means that they are unable to make a specific decision at the time it needs to be made. (Department of Constitutional Affairs 2007: 42)

The test that someone legally lacks capacity therefore has two components or steps. First, the patient must have some kind of mental or brain impairment, such as dementia, other mental health problem or confusion as a result of illness. Secondly, this impairment must be preventing their ability to make a particular decision at the time it is required. In Edith's case, she clearly has a progressive and longstanding impairment in her brain caused by multi-infarct dementia. In addition, she has a chest infection which may be causing additional cognitive impairment at this time. This situation does not necessarily prevent her from making any decisions at all. It is likely that she is fully able to make decisions, for example about what to eat or wear, but she may not be able to make complex decisions that affect her overall well-being. Her decision-making capacity must be carefully assessed, rather than assumed.

Under the provisions of the Mental Capacity Act 2005, a person may only be regarded as unable to make a decision if they cannot:

- understand information about the decision to be made
- retain that information in their mind
- use or weigh that information as part of the decision-making process, or
- communicate their decision (by talking, using sign language or any other means). (Department of Constitutional Affairs 2007: 45)

It is good practice for the assessment of these stages of decision-making to be documented in the patient's notes so that if the assessment result is challenged at a later date it can be justified.

The responsibility to assess mental capacity usually lies with the professional involved with the patient, and depends on the particular decision which is needed at the time. For example, if the decision is whether or not a patient is able to consent to having a bed bath, the responsibility for assessing their capacity to consent to that care is with the nurse or carer involved. In the case of Edith, responsibility for assessing Edith's ability to decide whether or not to take antibiotics lies with the prescribing GP, Dr Cooper, as the professional proposing the treatment. Dr Cooper may seek and take into account the views of the multidisciplinary team, so Charlotte and Janet are likely to be involved in the assessment too. Figure 4.1 considers the issues involved when assessing Edith's capacity.

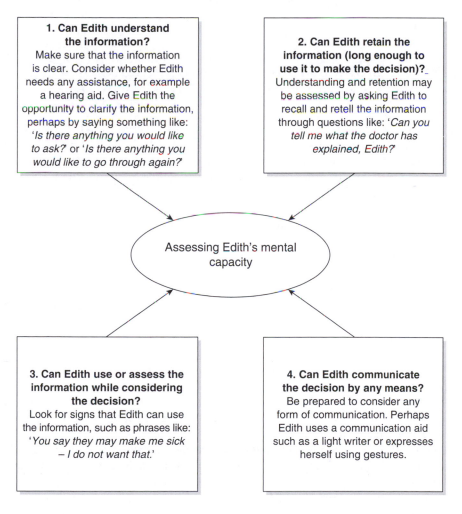

Figure 4.1   Assessing Edith's mental capacity to make a decision about whether or not to take antibiotics

Reflective question

Think of a situation which you have encountered in your practice in which you have wondered if a patient has the ability to make an important decision. This may be a decision that you were faced with, or one in which you were involved as part of the multidisciplinary team.

Consider each of the four points in Figure 4.1 and write a short paragraph outlining the patient's ability to undertake each step.

Can you reach a reasoned judgement of the patient's mental capacity or lack of it, and document it accordingly considering all four points?

How decisions are made regarding care of people who cannot express their own wishes

While it is important to start from the principle that everyone has the capacity to make decisions, for patients who have been assessed as lacking the capacity to make a decision at the time required, then the decision must be made on their behalf and in their best interests. In order to determine which course of action is in the patient's best interests the decision-maker should:

- Encourage the participation of the patient in making the decision in so far as he or she is able to participate.
- Identify all relevant circumstances, i.e. aspects that would be taken into account by the patient if they were making the decision.
- Find out the person's views. These may be articulated by someone who knows the patient, may have been previously written down, or perhaps expressed in their behaviour, such as being a member of a particular faith, culture or interest group.
- Avoid discrimination and assumption about what is in someone's best interest, e.g. on the basis of age.
- Assess whether the person might regain capacity and therefore whether waiting until the patient can make the decision themselves would be in their best interest.
- If the decision concerns life-sustaining treatment, decision-makers should not be motivated in any way by a desire to bring about the person's death, or make assumptions about the person's quality of life.
- Consult others. Best-interest decisions are best made in consultation with others who are involved in the patient's care and welfare, such as the multidisciplinary team, family and friends.
- Avoid restricting the person's rights.

This section is based on Chapter 5 of the Code of Practice relating to the Mental Capacity Act 2005 (Department of Constitutional Affairs 2007), which should be consulted if more information is required.

The person making a decision on behalf of someone who lacks capacity is required to weigh up all of these factors in order to establish what is in the person's best interests. The decision-maker should document the consideration of each in the patient's records, so that it is transparent to all and justifiable at a later date if required.

Reflective question

Dr Cooper considers that Edith lacks the capacity to make this decision though she is able to express her dislike of taking antibiotics. He turns next to consider whether antibiotic therapy is in Edith's best interest and asks Charlotte for her thoughts.

If you were in Charlotte's situation, how would you respond to Dr Cooper?

There are a number of issues to consider when making a decision about whether antibiotic treatment is in Edith's best interests. Figure 4.2 illustrates the issues Dr Cooper should consider. Charlotte, as part of the nursing team caring for Edith on a daily basis, has an important contribution to make to the process. It would be particularly important for Charlotte to inform Dr Cooper that she had been told that her daughter Sarah had 'legal responsibility'. Ideally, the nursing home should be aware of any such provision. If not, Charlotte should explore this comment further, perhaps contacting Sarah to clarify the position. Dr Cooper needs any information that might illuminate Edith's personal views, accurate information about her current clinical condition, including both the symptoms she is experiencing and her response to comfort-enhancing measures such as paracetamol. Sound nursing information of this type has a huge influence on clinical decision-making. Remember that Dr Cooper may have had limited recent contact with Edith and her family, and will be reliant on nursing home staff for this information.

Reflective question

Nurses frequently see themselves as the patient's advocate in difficult situations. What would acting as the patient's advocate mean to you if you were in Charlotte's situation?

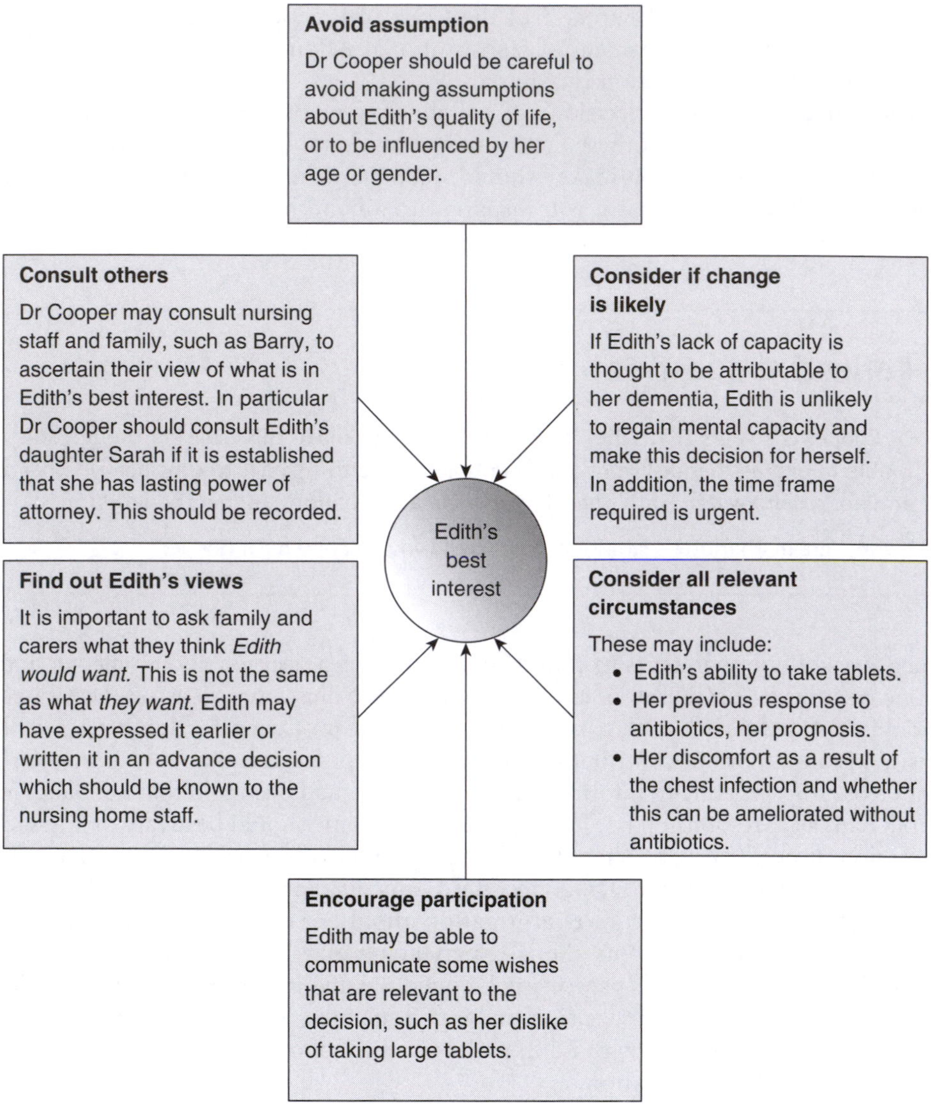

Avoid assumption

Dr Cooper should be careful to avoid making assumptions about Edith's quality of life, or to be influenced by her age or gender.

Consult others

Dr Cooper may consult nursing staff and family, such as Barry, to ascertain their view of what is in Edith's best interest. In particular Dr Cooper should consult Edith's daughter Sarah if it is established that she has lasting power of attorney. This should be recorded.

Consider if change is likely

If Edith's lack of capacity is thought to be attributable to her dementia, Edith is unlikely to regain mental capacity and make this decision for herself. In addition, the time frame required is urgent.

Find out Edith's views

It is important to ask family and carers what they think *Edith would want*. This is not the same as what *they want*. Edith may have expressed it earlier or written it in an advance decision which should be known to the nursing home staff.

Edith's best interest

Consider all relevant circumstances

These may include:
- Edith's ability to take tablets.
- Her previous response to antibiotics, her prognosis.
- Her discomfort as a result of the chest infection and whether this can be ameliorated without antibiotics.

Encourage participation

Edith may be able to communicate some wishes that are relevant to the decision, such as her dislike of taking large tablets.

Figure 4.2   Making a decision in Edith's best interests

Action point

Faced with making difficult decisions in patients' best interests, it is tempting to consider what *we* would want if we were faced with the same situation. We tend to imagine that patients would want the same as we would want for ourselves or our loved ones. While this is an understandable response, be aware that people make valid choices which may be different from your own. Try to focus on what *they* would want, regardless of your own ideas.

How people may influence decisions that may be made about them if they lose capacity in the future

The Mental Capacity Act 2005 provides the means for people with capacity to make provision for decision-making about themselves should they lose capacity to do so in the future.

Lasting Powers of Attorney

Under the provisions of the Mental Capacity Act 2005, people may appoint attorneys who can make decisions for them if, in the future, they lack the capacity to make decisions themselves. Any decisions made must be in the best interests of the person concerned. Lasting Powers of Attorney (LPAs) can be set up, both for health and welfare, and for property and financial matters. It is the former that is relevant to health care decisions.

Health and welfare attorneys can make a range of decisions including those relating to general care, consent to examinations, treatment and complaints. Persons making an LPA may also use it to specify the sort of decisions their attorney can make. To be valid, an LPA must be registered with the Office of the Public Guardian (OPG). Provided that an attorney's decisions are in the patient's best interest, they then carry the same authority as if they were those of the patient. It is vital that nurses are aware when valid LPAs exist for their patients, and that they record this, together with details of how to contact the attorney if this becomes necessary.

The nursing home in which Edith resides should be aware of her LPA. Knowing the significance of LPAs, Charlotte may be able to clarify Barry's comment that his sister has 'legal resposibilty' and explore this further.

Advance decision to refuse treatment

An additional way that the Mental Capacity Act 2005 enables individuals with mental capacity to influence decisions about their future care is through an 'advance decision to refuse treatment'. Adults over 18 years of age can make an advance decision to refuse a specific treatment that they may need in the future, should they lack the capacity to make that decision at that time. Valid advance decisions are legally binding, carrying the same legal status as a decision made by someone who has the capacity to make the decision at the time (Department of Constitutional Affairs 2007).

For an advance decision to be valid, the conditions set out in the Code of Practice (Department of Constitutional Affairs 2007) must be met. These conditions include that:

- the patient must not be able to make the decision at the time it needs to be made;
- it must apply to the specific situation/decision in question;
- it must be signed by the patient and witnessed. If a person is unable to sign, they can direct another to do it on their behalf as long as this is witnessed and signed by a third party;
- if the treatment in question is potentially life sustaining/prolonging, the advance decision must state 'even if my life is at risk'.

Action point

Look at the sample advance decision below. Which three aspects of it are important to ensure its validity?

Advance decision

I, Elsie Clarke of 17 Yeats Close, declare that should my breast cancer illness advance to the extent that I am unable to communicate decisions about my care in the future, I would not like to be given treatment to prolong my life, such as tube feeding or heart resuscitation even if my life is at risk.

Signed by Elsie Clarke 12 March 2009

Witnessed by Michael Baters (Neighbour) 12 March 2009

The important aspects are that it is signed and witnessed, and that it states 'even if my life is at risk'.

It is vital that health care professionals are aware of the existence of advance decisions to refuse treatments and that they are documented. Health care professionals may be involved in advising patients of the opportunity to make an advance decision while they have capacity. Returning to the case study, it appears that Edith did not make a valid advance decision refusing antibiotics, but if she had, it would have carried the same legal weight as if she had refused antibiotics at the time.

The role of health care students in end-of-life care decision-making

Like Charlotte, health care students are often involved in difficult decision-making. Difficult decisions, by their nature, can be daunting. In Edith's case, the consequences of deciding not to treat her infection with antibiotics may seem overwhelming. However, it is important to appreciate that such decisions are made in consultation with patients, their families and a wide health care team, and are guided by ethical principles and governed by legislation. Under the supervision of mentors, students like Charlotte can contribute to difficult ethical decision-making on the same basis as all members of the health care team.

Action point

As part of your learning, notice how decisions are made and documented. Relevant information you may observe may include:

- Expression of preference by the patient
- Preferences of the family
- Supporting patients to understand the choices they face and to communicate their decisions
- Assessment of capacity
- Best interest decisions

Returning to Edith's case

Dr Cooper made a careful assessment of Edith's situation. On learning that Edith had appointed Sarah as a health and welfare attorney, Dr Cooper discussed the situation with her.

Dr Cooper established that Sarah had indeed a valid health and welfare LPA for Edith, and was specifically authorised to refuse life-sustaining treatment on her behalf. Sarah said that when Edith was first diagnosed with dementia, she had discussed her wishes for her future care with Sarah. Edith had recalled that her own mother had not wished to be kept alive when life was no longer enjoyable. She trusted Sarah to make that judgement if she became in that position. Sarah now feels that Edith would not wish to be hospitalised and take further oral antibiotics again if her symptoms can be controlled in other ways.

Appreciating that Sarah is acting in Edith's best interests, Dr Cooper agrees to treat Edith's infection palliatively within the nursing home.

Summary

This chapter has discussed the influence of key ethical principles in health care, and is based on the Mental Capacity Act 2005 Code of Practice (Department of Constitutional Affairs 2007). Understanding these areas is vital in order to enable patients to make choices and, when patients are unable to do this, make ethical decisions on their behalf. Key points to remember when faced with difficult decisions at the end of a patient's life are:

- Always consider who is the right person to make the decision.
- Consider whether a patient needs information, practical assistance or support in decision-making.
- If, despite all support, they remain unable to make the decision, consider whether they lack the capacity. This should be formally assessed and documented.
- If patients lack capacity to make one decision, remember they may be able to make other decisions.
- Any decision made on behalf of a patient who lacks capacity must be made on the basis of his or her best interests. This applies both to decisions made by a clinician responsible for care or treatment, and to decisions made on the patient's behalf by a properly appointed attorney.

Further reading

NHS End of Life Care Programme and the National Council for Palliative Care (2008) *Advance Decisions to RefuseTreatment – A Guide for Health and Social Care Professionals* [online]. Available at: www.endoflifecare.nhs.uk/eolc/files/NHS-EoLC_ADRT_Sep2008.pdf [accessed 30 April 2012].
This helpful publication explains advance decisions to refuse treatment within the Mental Capacity Act 2005.

National End of Life Care Programme (2011) *Capacity, Care Planning and Advance Care Planning in Life Limiting Illness – A Guide for Health and Social Care Staff.* [online]. Available at: www.endoflifecareforadults.nhs.uk/assets/downloads/ACP_booklet_2011_Final_1.pdf [accessed 1 May 2012].
This useful document, written under the End of Life Care Programme, explains issues of assessment of capacity and care planning in patients facing the end of their lives.

General Medical Council (GMC) (2010*) Treatment and Care towards the End of Life: Good Practice in Decision-Making.* London: GMC [online]. Available at: www.gmc-uk.org/static/documents/content/End_of_life.pdf [accessed 1 May 2012].
While this publication has been written for doctors, it is very useful in explaining their role and the process of ethical decision-making.

References

Beauchamp, T.L. and Childress, J.F. (2001) *Principles of Biomedical Ethics* (5th edn). Oxford: Oxford University Press.

Chater, K. and Tsai, C. (2008) 'Palliative care in a multicultural society: a challenge for western ethics', *Australian Journal of Advanced Nursing*, 26(2): 95–100.

Department of Constitutional Affairs (2007) *The Mental Capacity Act 2005: Code of Practice.* London: The Stationery Office. Available online at: http://webarchive.nationalarchives.gov. uk/+/http://www.dca.gov.uk/legal-policy/mental-capacity/mca-cp.pdf [accessed 30 April 2012].

Department of Health (2008) *The End of Life Care Strategy.* London: DH.

Griffin, R. and Tengnah, C. (2010) *Law and Professional Issues in Nursing* (2nd edn). Exeter: Learning Matters.

Nightingale, F. (1863) *Notes on Hospitals.* London: Longman, Green, Longman, Roberts and Green.

Pettifer, A., Cooper, J. and Munday, D. (2007) 'Teaching inter-professional teamwork in palliative care – a values-based approach', *Journal of Palliative Care*, 23(4): 280–5.

Randall, F. and Downie, R.S. (2001) *Palliative Care Ethics: A Companion for All Specialities* (2nd edn). Oxford: Oxford Medical Publications.

Thoresen, L. (2003) 'A reflection on Cicely Saunders' views on a good death through the philosophy of Charles Taylor', *International Journal of Palliative Care Nursing*, 9(1): 19–23.

Thorns, A. (1998) 'Ethics: a review of the doctrine of double effect', *European Journal of Palliative Care*, 5(4): 117–20.

UK Parliament (2005) *The Mental Capacity Act 2005* [Act of Parliament]. London: The Stationery Office. Available online at: www.legislation.gov.uk/ukpga/2005/9/pdfs/ ukpga_20050009_en.pdf [accessed 30 April 2012].

CHAPTER 5

Calling in the palliative care team

Joanna De Souza

This chapter will explore:

- The different levels of palliative care
- Making specialist palliative care referrals
- Involving the family as part of the care team
- Making use of the multidisciplinary specialist palliative care team
- When professionals have different views on how a patient should be cared for

Introduction

When it becomes clear that a patient is nearing the end of life, it can raise a feeling of anxiety in us as professionals, about what the patient's needs may be and that we will not be able to meet them all. It is common that when a decision is made that a patient will have no further curative treatment, someone will suggest that a referral is made to the specialist palliative care team. This chapter will explore how this may be done appropriately.

Increasingly, although the understanding of what palliative care as an approach has to offer patients, patients are remaining under acute teams having what we call active treatment. When dealing with patients whose conditions cannot be cured, the end-of-life care strategy offers the 'surprise question' – *Would you be surprised if this patient were to die within the next six months to a year?* If the answer to this question is no, then it may be appropriate to progress to taking a palliative approach.

The following case study illustrates a situation where a patient is facing an end-of-life decision and their palliative care needs are likely to increase in the near future. In this case, the transition into the dying phase is likely to be rapid, so this patient and family may have a high level of psychological and physical needs ahead.

Bert

Bert Williams, an 80 year-old gentleman, developed acute and then chronic renal failure following a road traffic accident 15 years ago. The accident damaged one kidney through trauma and the second kidney due to the stress placed upon it from the accident and subsequent period of dehydration. Following a short period on haemodialysis, he received a donor kidney which functioned well, but over the last couple of years the function has been deteriorating and he has again required haemodialysis. Bert also has a history of cardiac failure and his cardiac function has been deteriorating over the past year. He has been admitted to the ward with a urinary tract infection.

On admission he was quite confused and had low-grade pyrexia, and his glomerular filtration rate was 10ml/min/1.73m². However, following a course of antibiotics, his confusion has resolved though his condition remains poor. The doctors have decided that Bert is unlikely to benefit from continued haemodialysis. However, they are awaiting the results of some tests before discussing this with him. Following the ward round, you are relieved when the doctors suggest that you or your mentor should contact the palliative care team and ask if they can come and see Bert.

Looking at the situation with Bert, Lamping et al. (2000) found that 50% of all patients over the age of 80 had died within a year of starting dialysis, compared with 20% who started between the ages of 70 and 74. Dialysis is a demanding and arduous treatment, particularly in elderly people (Noble and Lewis 2008), so assisting people to make informed decisions about commencing or continuing such treatments is an important part of supportive care.

Reflective question

Once an end-of-life situation has been identified, nurses will often choose to call in the palliative care team immediately. What anxieties does this situation create for you and what do you hope the palliative care team will be able to do?

What can the palliative care team do?

When we consider Bert's needs, several of the symptoms he is experiencing are things that we may deal with every day as part of normal nursing care. What sometimes makes the care of a patient who is at the end of life difficult is the extent of the problems or symptoms and also the complexity of having multiple severe symptoms.

In many instances care can be provided by the health care team that is most involved with the patient. In Bert's case, the renal team and his own GP will have been offering some of this care already as his condition deteriorated. However, when there are difficult decisions that involve end-of-life care, and issues such as ceasing active treatments, specialist teams can offer valuable support to the generalist team, the patient and the family.

The specialised palliative care team may also be able to help the general health care team in their discussions with Bert and his family about where Bert would like to be cared for as he comes to the end of his life. In situations where someone close to the end of life would like to go home to die, decisions will need to be made quickly and community services set up. This is discussed more fully in Chapter 7. Specialist teams often play a large role in facilitating early discharge for patients at the end of life. This increased involvement may be because they have established links with community teams and resources and so can facilitate quick and effective discharges when there are complex needs to consider. For example, someone at the end of life may need a hospital bed, oxygen at home and night sitters to be arranged very quickly to ensure they remain well enough to get home before they die.

What this means for the patient

For Bert, once his new kidney started failing and it was not going to be appropriate to give him another, a palliative approach would be required. This would include ensuring that Bert had as much information as possible about his condition to allow him to start making decisions about what interventions would enable him to achieve the best quality of life for himself and his family. Some patients are keen to have all the active treatment they can, others prefer to wind down on active treatment and maximise their time at home. A true palliative approach is being able to support a patient while they make these decisions and to provide time to talk over the options with them and plan for the future.

Reflective questions

If you were looking after Bert, how do you think you might start a conversation with him about his care? What do you feel you would want to know before you had that conversation?

For many patients there is a particular time when decisions are made to discontinue significant interventions. With cancer patients this may be chemotherapy and with others it may be other interventions, such as regular blood transfusions. These are always complex decisions and ones where family members may feel differently from each other or even to the patient. Being able to facilitate family discussions about how this may affect the patient in the days to come and to explore any worries different people may have at this stage is a very important task for the multidisciplinary team.

Bert, once he has stopped having interventions such as dialysis, will deteriorate quickly. In some ways with renal failure patients, this makes the decision-making particularly complex. However, his terminal care is more predictable than in other conditions where treatment may have been stopped and of a short duration, usually no more than 10 days.

The different levels of palliative care

In 1996, the NHS Executive produced a model which divided palliative care into three tiers:

1   Palliative care approach
2   Palliative interventions
3   Specialist palliative care.

This model was devised to help health care professionals recognise their own responsibilities to their patients nearing the end of life, but also to help health care teams decide when it is appropriate to refer to specialist palliative care teams. Similarly, the International Association for Hospice and Palliative Care (IAHPC) describe these in their manual of palliative care as:

- **palliative care principles**, which apply to all care, whatever the disease suffered by a patient and can be offered by health care professionals.
- **palliative techniques or therapies**, which include medical procedures and surgical therapies, for example placing a stenting, removing acitic fluid by paracentesis, or radiotherapy, all for symptom control measures but the interventions are offered to the patient often earlier on in their disease trajectory without the whole team being involved.
- **specialist palliative care**, where there are complex palliative care needs which require the whole specialist team to be involved in the care (Doyle and Woodruff 2008).

The palliative care approach

The history of this approach is discussed in Chapter 1. It had its origins in the 1960s, driven by the work of Dame Cicely Saunders and others such as Professor John Hinton, who recognised that there was a need for active involvement in end-of-life care to facilitate better symptom control and healthy psychosocial adjustment.

The approach is encapsulated by the definition provided by the World Health Organisation:

> Palliative care is defined as an approach that focuses on the quality of life of patients and their families with life-threatening illness, through the prevention and relief of suffering facilitated by appropriate early identification and evidence-based assessment with the treatment of both physical and psychosocial issues. (WHO 2012)

In 2004, the National Institute for Clinical Excellence (NICE 2004) produced the *Supportive Care Guidelines* which contained recommendations about issues such as appropriate delivery of diagnosis, effective multidisciplinary care, including the appointment of a key worker, use of tools such as the Gold Standards Framework, end-of-life care pathways and access to specialist services when required. At the time, these recommendations related specifically to cancer patients, but in the *End of Life Care Strategy* (Department of Health 2008) it is recommended that all health care professionals should be using this approach when working with all who face death, regardless of diagnosis.

It is widely debated in the literature that this approach is simply one of good health care that incorporates all the central tenets of ethically sound care, such as promoting patient autonomy and decision-making, as has been discussed in Chapter 4.

Palliative interventions

Palliative care interventions are described as non-curative treatments aimed at relieving symptoms or improving quality of life by specialists outside palliative care. They include the use of palliative chemotherapy, radiotherapy and surgery, particularly anaesthetic procedures. Increasingly, they also involve the use of rehabilitation therapists. These interventions almost inevitably require the input of specialist practitioners but it may be only for an advisory meeting or for a fixed period of time that the patient receives such intervention. In addition, it would often involve input from a specific member of the specialist team rather than the whole team involvement.

Specialist palliative care

When a patient has a complex set of problems that require specialist input, such as advanced cancer patients with complex pain needs, or chronic obstructive pulmonary disease (COPD) patients with complex breathing difficulties, it can be useful to call in a specialist team to give advice on how to manage these problems.

Specialist palliative care is given by a multi-professional team who have undergone recognised specialist palliative care training (Clinical Standards Board for Scotland 2002). For our patient, Bert, there may be two specialist teams involved:

the hospital-based palliative care team, who may get involved to deal with immediate symptom control and to liaise around discharge, and the community-based palliative care team, who will be on hand to advise the community health team and to work with Bert and the family once Bert has gone home.

In his work looking at professional involvement in palliative medicine, Gannon (2008) explores the potential benefits that health care professionals (HCPs) can facilitate. These are outlined below:

- Accurate information to aid treatment choices
- Active treatment of underlying disease
- Relief from symptoms
- Reassurance and inspiring confidence
- Respecting patient autonomy
- Empowerment of patients
- Provision of emotional support
- Mobilisation of other appropriate disciplines
- Lightening the burden placed on patients and relatives
- Bereavement support
- Potential for future improvements in the care of the dying

Although some of these aspects may fit into a palliative care approach, with patients with complex needs, or where the patient is transferring between services, it is helpful to have this level of competency, which is often held by the specialist team.

Gannon also offers an important warning about how we can over-medicalise death and how health care professionals can undermine patient choice and autonomy through paternalistic practice and a loss of focus on the aims of the palliative care interventions. He is concerned about the increasing institutionalisation of death as a result of the development of knowledge and technology, which leads to an increased exposure to drugs and investigations and an additional burden of how and when to stop treatments. He warned that we run the risk of abusing the privileged position we hold as health care professionals.

Reflective questions

Think of a patient you have looked after with long-term illness who you would consider to be in their last year of life:

Do you feel that the care being taken was following the palliative care approach?

1 Why do you think that was?
2 When a referral was made to the specialist palliative care team, what was it for?
3 Having considered the definition above, do you feel it was necessary at that point to involve the specialist team?

Nearing the end of life

Bert has reached the fifth stage of chronic kidney disease with his glomerular filtration rate (GFR) running at less than 15, which is an indicator that he has very little kidney function remaining. He will increasingly experience the symptoms of renal failure. However, the onset is gradual and usually accompanied by lethargy and sleepiness so for many patients death is quite gentle.

Normally, the kidney maintains the body's fluid balance by a complex relationship between hormone production and secretion, electrolyte balance, and waste-product elimination. In renal failure, these functions are not performed and complications, such as uraemia, anaemia, hyperkalemia, and hypertension occur quite rapidly in the absence of any renal function. Ureamia occurs as the levels of urea build up in his blood stream. Patients may experience nausea and vomiting, fatigue, weight loss, muscle cramps, puritis (itching), and slowly increasing confusion and coma as a result. As anaemia sets in, patients will have problems with coagulation and as well as symptoms of anaemia, weakness and breathlessness, they may experience nose bleeds or gingivitis or bleeding gums. As renal function declines, the nephron is unable to excrete the potassium ions, hyperkalemia results with a corresponding effect of raising the blood pressure and causing cardiac arrhythmias.

Noble, an experienced renal nurse, discussed the importance of opening up discussion with patients for whom dialysis may not be beneficial (Noble and Lewis 2008). At this stage it is important for both patients and their families to discuss the implications of the decisions that have to be made. This will give them space to ask the questions they may have, and will also allow them to grieve for the losses that they will feel under these circumstances. It is the challenge of doing this that is sometimes felt to require the specialist communication skills of a palliative care team. In reality, many experienced nurses and other multidisciplinary team members working in the speciality may be able to have this discussion in a more helpful way for their patients, as they have already built up a relationship with them and they have an in-depth understanding of the symptoms the patient may experience.

Action point

When you are looking after a patient for whom these types of decisions are being made, try to ensure that you are present for these discussions. Starting to engage with them as you work with patients facing all types of losses is the best preparation for developing your confidence in being able to promote these types of discussions with patients and families.

Prior to discharge, it will be important to explain to Bert's family what sort of symptoms he may experience so that they can go home with some suitable symptom control measures to use. The nurse can explain that he will become increasingly sleepy and may experience some nausea and itchiness, for which he will be sent home with a low dose of an antiemetic. Patients with impaired renal function eliminate medications very slowly so it is important to reduce standard doses in discussion with the renal team.

Bert will also be given some emollients to use to preserve his skin integrity and ease the discomfort of his itching, and also some antihistamine for use if it disturbs him at night. Ceasing his dialysis will also lead him to retain fluids and produce minimal amounts of urine. The renal team will need to manage his diuretics and give advice on diet as he will need to avoid salty or sugary foods and to maintain a low fluid intake. This build-up of fluid and toxins can result in pain and discomfort. Murtagh et al. (2007) offer a useful discussion of symptom control in this group of patients.

Bert is in a complex situation because of his underlying disease. The end stages of Bert's disease may be fairly rapid as he has no renal function. The end-of-life trajectory for renal patients is often a long series of peaks and troughs with a sharp decline at the end. Thus Bert's symptoms may change quickly and could be severe. In addition, both he and his family will need to adjust quickly to his deterioration and ensuing death. In this case, because of the time factors, it may be appropriate to call in the specialist palliative care team to look at support for his family, particularly if Bert wishes to die at home.

Making specialist palliative care referrals

Deciding when to refer to specialist palliative care teams is a matter under some debate. A summit looking at delivering better end-of-life care (Addicott and Ashton 2010) recognised the need to develop triggers for individual conditions that may help professionals have more clarity about when it is appropriate to refer to a specialist team. Many of the current models are based on an outdated cancer model from the time when many cancers had a predictable downward trajectory. Having decided to involve the specialist palliative care team, it is important to offer them as accurate a referral as possible so that they are aware of the precise areas of care in which the team is seeking help and guidance.

Reflective questions

Thinking about the patients you have looked after who were at the end of life, how did their underlying condition affect the last part of their life journey (trajectory)?

How did the different trajectories influence the way their care was planned and delivered?

When making a referral for Bert and his family to a specialist team, it is important to indicate that you are referring him because you are expecting sudden deterioration. He is no longer receiving dialysis so has a very limited prognosis and with imminent need for symptom control and psychological support in this rapidly changing situation.

Involving the family as part of the care team

Communication with any family when one of their members is facing death is an essential part of patient care and allows them to be and feel more involved in the care. Monroe and Oliviere (2009) illustrate that, as professionals, we can choose the way in which we view families. We can see them as entities separate from the patient who need an individual type of care, or we can view them as an integral part of the patient's care and care for the patient and family as a system. Their work demonstrates the co-dependency that exists between patients and their families (or social networks). They also discuss how families are not always carers or drift in and out of the caregiving role at different times in the illness journey.

If we are to see Bert and his family as a system, then we need to include them in the information-giving and allow them to participate in the decision-making that will involve them, such as discharge planning, giving them an opportunity to express the fears and concerns they may have. Monroe and Olivere (2009) offer a useful model for meeting with families. They discuss the importance of using family meetings to help people normalise the situation they find themselves in, that is, to offer assurance that the difficulties they are having are shared by other families facing these types of situation. They remind us that people will have worries about how they will cope, and they can perhaps feel empowered by being given information about how they might deal with the problems that may occur. Lastly, they stress the importance of working with families to help and encourage them to change some of the ways in which the family operates and the expectations they may have of family life in light of their new reality of their loved one's abilities to fulfil and participate in their traditional roles.

Making Use of the Multidisciplinary Specialist Palliative Care Team

The health care team is designed to provide a rich resource for meeting the complex needs of ill health. By working together, a multidisciplinary team approach has been shown to improve clinical outcomes and quality of life (NHS Improvement 2012). In end-of-life care individual roles are often less defined than in more acute areas of care, with different members of the team undertaking different roles depending on their relationships with patients and families. The National End of Life Care Programme has developed core competencies in end-of-life care (NELCP 2009) that allow for this blurring of role boundaries.

Chapter 1 looks at the development of palliative and end-of-life care as specialist disciplines in medicine and nursing, which represent the largest groups of health care professionals involved. However, as palliative care has emerged as a speciality, specialist roles within many of the health care professions have developed. Today many specialist palliative care teams include social workers, occupational therapists, physiotherapists and other therapists, including art and music therapists and spiritual councillors such as chaplains. An example of one of these specialist roles is that of the palliative care social workers.

Traditionally, social work has been seen as an expression of humanitarianism, but it has also been condemned as an agent of social control, being associated with mainly poor and disadvantaged people (Beresford et al. 2007). However, over the past 30 years, social work in palliative care has become a speciality of its own. The role is defined by the Association of Palliative Care Social Workers (APCSW 2012) as one that offers a range of support to patients and families, including practical help, advice around social issues such as finance and housing, help in accessing other services, and counselling and support. This support includes bereavement work. Their main aim is to see people as a whole and not as set of problems, to understand the connections of their lives and to act, rather than ignore, the constraints they experience in society.

The aim is that all the different professionals bring their range of skills and knowledge to the difficult tasks involved in delivering effective end-of-life care. They also allow decision-making and care planning to take a holistic approach.

As a more junior member of the health care team, it is often very difficult to understand and be a part of the decisions that are made about the care plan for a patient you are involved with. Alternatively, as you have slightly fewer demands on your time, you may have an opportunity to be present more often when other professionals see and discuss things with your patient. You may then find yourself caught between the views of the different HCPs looking after the patient. Developing a good relationship with all members of the health care team of which you are a part is the first step to being able to participate in and contribute to care discussions.

Communication is often the key factor in opposing views. Teams which have a culture of open conversation and which facilitate opportunities for discussion between all the members of the team caring for a patient will often be able to discuss the rationale for the treatment decisions they wish to make. It is important to be as informed as possible about the patient's situation but also to be able to explore the ideology behind the views of others when these are different from your own or from that of one professional group. Involving the patient in these decisions whenever possible can often help to guide the situation.

Bert (2)

CASE STUDY

Bert and his wife, Iris, decided that he would now like to stop treatment as he was finding it increasingly difficult to come to the hospital for dialysis. He has been feeling increasingly unwell and knew he would not be able to tolerate another transplant. Bert had previously thought about what he would want when he reached this stage before his first transplant. Their daughter Olwen has flown over from her home in Ireland to

(Continued)

(Continued)

be with her parents. She was quite upset when she first arrived on the ward. You sat in on a discussion with your mentor and Olwen as she explained what to expect.

She explained that although Bert had stopped his dialysis it was difficult to predict the exact amount of time he had left. She was able to let her know that it would be days and weeks rather than months.

The family were referred to the district nurses for help with physical care and were encouraged to consider having a hospital bed in the house so that it would be easier to position Bert when he became less able to move himself. Bert, Olwen and Iris remained anxious about the decision they were making, but were aware that the HCPs in the community would be visiting and were contactable at any time. They were also aware that the medical team had spoken to their GP and he too would be visiting soon. Iris and Olwen were encouraged to share Bert's care plan with any HCPs who attended Bert at home so that the decisions that had been made about his care could be carried out.

About 10 days after his discharge, the ward received a card from Iris and Olwen explaining that Bert had died peacefully at home and they were in the process of planning his funeral. Although it had been hard, they were grateful to the ward team for the sensitive way in which Bert's care had been managed.

Reflective question

Enabling a patient to make decisions about their care can be a very rewarding experience. However, when patients are discharged or transferred we do not always know what happens to them.

If you look after someone who dies peacefully or recovers from a long-term illness for which they have been receiving a significant amount of their care from another health care professional, would you consider contacting them to let them know the patient's outcome?

Supporting patients and families when caring for people at the end of life in their own homes is an area in which specialist palliative care teams have played a major role. However, Nyatanga (2008) reminds us that for some patients and their families being able to die at home and in control of their own circumstances, such as in the case of Bert, is achieved in increasingly fewer situations due to our medical ability to continually offer more life-sustaining treatments. As health care professionals, we can be anxious about our own need to treat a patient's every complaint/symptom to the point of preventing them from achieving their own goals of a good death.

Specialist palliative care teams often come skilled in managing these types of anxieties and the staff who work in them carry the confidence of knowing what is possible and what can be achieved. This can influence the medical team's decisions in a way that can sometimes be difficult for the nursing teams at ward level.

When professionals have different views on how a patient should be cared for

Conflicting views about when to take on a palliative care approach and when to involve a specialist palliative care team continue to abound. Merryn Gott et al. (2001), in their study of nurses and doctors, explore some of these differences. Their study was interesting because it established that patients with non-cancer diagnoses were more likely to be picked up by nurses (rather than by the medical staff) as having palliative care needs. In part this is due to the complexity of diagnosing the end stage of dying in some conditions, and an assumption by some professionals that palliative care is only about withdrawing interventions; it is an either/or situation where one must make a decision to either be offering active interventionist care or withdraw active care, but it also raises questions about what it means to have palliative care needs. However, it is hoped that by considering end of life as a stage (see Chapter 1) rather than simply the last weeks of life, a better sense of collaboration will be established between specialist palliative care teams and other teams working in acute settings. Open communication and an ability to participate fully in all patient care planning is an important aim for the multi-professional team in all areas.

Summary

The key points to remember when deciding when to call in the palliative care team are:

- To establish what the patient's and family's needs are at the time.
- To establish early on a palliative care approach and to initiate some of the difficult conversations and comfort measures of care.
- To ascertain whether the patient and their family have complex palliative care needs and, having called in the specialist team, to work with them to achieve optimum end-of-life care for your patients.

Further reading

The Gold Standards Framework website is a useful resource to explore. The approach, initially developed for community teams, is now being implemented in inpatient settings and offers a great approach for teamworking: www.goldstandardsframework.org.uk.

Peter Speck, a health care chaplain and researcher, has edited this useful book, which also touches on aspects of teamwork that can be difficult: Peter Speck (ed.) (2006) *Teamwork in Palliative Care. Fulfilling or Frustrating? Looking at the Role of Teamwork and Some of the Important Aspects of it in Palliative Care*. Oxford: Oxford University Press.

Another book that offers some valuable insights into how to work effectively alongside our patients' lay carers, who in many situations provide the major part of the care they require, is: Peter Hudson and Sheila Payne (eds) (2009) *Family Carers in Palliative Care: A Guide for Health and Social Care Professionals*. Oxford: Oxford University Press.

References

Addicott, R. and Ashton, R. (2010) *Delivering Better Care at End of Life: The Next Steps*. Report from the Sir Roger Bannister Health Summit, November 2009. London: Kings Fund, UK.

APCSW (2012) Association of Palliaitve Care Social Workers [online]. Available at: www.apcsw.org.uk [accessed 11 September 2012].

Beresford, P., Adshead, L. and Croft, S. (2007) *Palliative Care, Social Work and Service Users: Making Life Possible*. London: Jessica Kingsley.

Clinical Standards Board for Scotland (2002) *Clinical Standards for Specialist Palliative Care*. Edinburgh: CSBS.

Department of Health (2008) *The End of Life Care Strategy*. London: Department of Health.

Department of Health Renal NSF Team and Marie Curie Palliative Care Institute (2008) *Guidelines for LCP Prescribing in Advanced Chronic Kidney Disease* [online]. Available at: www.renal.org/.../NationalLCPRenalSymptomControlGuideline [accessed 11 September 2012].

Doyle, D. and Woodruff, R. (2008) *The IAHPC Manual of Palliative Care* (2nd edn). IAHPC Press. Available online at: www.hospicecare.com/manual/IAHPCmanual.htm [accessed 25 May 2012].

Gannon, G. (2008) 'An overview of the medicalisation of death', Chapter 4 in B. Nyatanga (ed.), *Why Is It So Difficult to Die?* London: Quay Books.

Lamping, D., Constantinovici, N., Roderick, P., Normand, C., Henderson, L., Harris, S., Brown, E., Gruen, R. and Victor, C. (2000) 'Clinical outcomes, quality of life and costs in a North Thames dialysis study of elderly people on dialysis: a prospective cohort study', *The Lancet*, 356: 1543–50.

Merryn Gott, C., Ahmedzai, S. and Wood, C. (2001) 'How many inpatients at an acute hospital have palliative care needs? Comparing the perspectives of medical and nursing staff', *Palliative Medicine*, 15(6): 451–60.

Monroe, B. and Oliviere, D. (2009) 'Communicating with family carers', Chapter 1 in P. Hudson and S. Payne (eds), *Family Carers in Palliative Care: A Guide for Health and Social Care Professionals*. Oxford: Oxford University Press.

Murtagh, F., Chai, M.O., Donohoe, P., Edmonds, P.M. and Higginson, I.J. (2007) 'The use of opioid analgesia in end-stage renal disease patients managed without dialysis: recommendations for practice', *Journal of Pain Palliative Care Pharmacotherapy*, 21(2): 5–16.

Murtagh, F., Murphy, E. and Sheerin, N. (2008) 'Illness trajectories: an important concept in the management of kidney failure', *Nephrology Dialysis Transplantation*, 23(12): 3746–8.

National Health Service (NHS) Executive (1996) *A Policy Framework for Commissioning Cancer Services: Palliative Care Services*. London: NHS Executive.

NHS Improvement (2012) NHS Improvement – Heart [online]. Available at: www.improvement.nhs.uk/heart/heartfailure/Home/HeartFailure.aspx [accessed 11 September 2012].

NELCP (2009) *Common Core Competences and Principles: A Guide for Health and Social Care Workers Working with Adults at the End of Life*. The National End of Life Care Programme. London: Department of Health / Skills for Care / Skills for Health.

NICE (2004) *Improving Supportive and Palliative care for adults with Cancer* [online]. London: National Institute for Clinical Excellence.

Noble, H. and Lewis, R. (2008) 'Assessing palliative care needs in end stage kidney disease', *Nursing Times*, 104(23): 26–7.

Nyatanga, B. (ed.) (2008) *Why Is It So Difficult to Die?* London: Quay Books.

Payne, S. (2010) 'White Paper on improving support for family carers in Palliative care: Part 1 Recommendations from the European Association for Palliative Care (EAPC) Task Force on Family Carers', *European Journal of Palliative Care*, 17(5): 238–45.

WHO (2012) *WHO Definition of Palliative Care* [online]. Available at: www.who.int/cancer/palliative/definition/en [accessed 11 September 2012].

CHAPTER 6

Managing physical symptoms

Joanna De Souza

This chapter will explore:

- The aims of symptom control at the end of life
- The common physical symptoms that cause distress at the end of life
- Assessing and managing symptoms

Introduction

Looking after someone who is uncomfortable or distressed is always difficult, particularly when you have given them all the medication they are prescribed and the symptoms don't go away. Often we are looking after patients in busy environments when there doesn't always seem to be time to ask someone more senior to come and give advice.

Good symptom control is one of the key features of palliative and end-of-life care. If we return to the definition of palliative care from the World Health Organisation, this states that: 'Palliative care is the relief of suffering facilitated by appropriate early identification and evidence-based assessment with the treatment of both physical and psychosocial issues' (WHO 2010). This reminds us that our main aim is to relieve suffering. That may be achieved by removing the cause of the symptoms, but often when working with patients at the end of life, removing the cause may actually result in more suffering than the symptom itself. We have discussed the issues around making a decision to stop pursuing curative treatments in Chapters 3 and 4.

The aims of symptom control at the end of life

The WHO definition also talks about using symptom control to help people live as actively as possible before death and to enhance the quality of their lives in ways which may also positively influence the course of illness. This reminds us that palliative and end-of-life care are not synonymous with terminal care and so we need to ensure that taking a palliative approach should not be seen primarily as a passive and withdrawing intervention (Yohannes 2007).

In a global resource, *The Palliative Care Toolkit* (Bond et al. 2008), the Worldwide Palliative Care Alliance, supported by Help the Hospices, base their symptom-control approach on three main principles or tasks. These are:

- **Task 1: Treat the treatable** – Establish what may be causing the symptom and treat it if possible and appropriately. For example, does your patient have an infection or a deep vein thrombosis that can be treated?
- **Task 2: Care for the patient** – The aim of symptom control at the end of life is to make the patient feel more comfortable. This must remain the focus of any interventions. Care needs to be taken to involve patients in their symptom control and to maintain patient dignity through the care offered.
- **Task 3: Prescribe palliative drugs** – Sometimes in end-of-life situations we may use medications in different ways and at different doses to achieve the desired effect. Concern about escalating doses and issues about dependence can result in under-dosage and reduced effectiveness.

This chapter aims to develop understanding of what these three tasks mean when you are involved with co-ordinating care for your patients.

The common physical symptoms that cause distress at the end of life

Solano, Gomes and Higginson (2006) compared the different end-of-life symptoms of people with advanced cancer, AIDS, heart disease, chronic obstructive pulmonary disease (COPD) and renal disease. They found a variety of symptom experiences, but the three most prevalent were pain, fatigue and breathlessness. A more recent study by Burt et al. (2010), which focused on older people dying from a variety of disorders, discovered that the three most common symptoms were pain, breathlessness and constipation.

The following case study illustrates a situation where a patient's symptoms are changing with the progression of her disease. We will use this example to explore the management of the common symptoms identified above.

Aarti

Mrs Shah (who likes to be called Aarti) is currently undergoing a course of palliative chemotherapy for her recurrent breast cancer. She has come in for her third course of treatment, so you have got to know her and her daughter quite well. She is very keen to finish the treatment. She is becoming increasingly breathless as she has active disease in her lungs and is finding it increasingly painful to move around because the cancer has spread to the bone (secondaries) in her spine and left arm. She arrives at the chemotherapy day unit to have her treatment. She is assisted by her daughter, who had to get a wheelchair at the front entrance as Aarti is finding it hard to walk very far due to breathlessness and pain. The unit is busy and you have been asked to settle Aarti in so she is ready to have her treatment.

Assessing and managing symptoms

It is always quite difficult to know how to address a patient's symptoms when you are in a busy environment and it is not necessarily easy to speak to them privately. However, it is important to remember that as Aarti is being treated as an outpatient, many of her interactions with health care professionals will be short. Aarti's arrival in a wheelchair offers you a good starting point for an enquiry into her symptoms, which have obviously progressed since her last visit.

We have already discussed the need for a holistic assessment in palliative care in Chapter 2 of this book. That chapter explores some of the assessment tools that have been developed within palliative care and, in particular, the PEPSI COLA *aide-mémoire* for holistic assessment. This chapter will look more specifically at some of the physical symptoms that patients may experience (i.e. the information that may fall in the P of PEPSI COLA).

Using comprehensive symptom assessment tools

Comprehensive structured symptom assessment tools can offer a useful form of initial screening to get a sense of what problems a patient has and their order of severity. Symptom assessment consists of collecting both objective and subjective information, for instance, both vital observations and also an account from the patient of the severity of the symptom. It is also important that assessment is an ongoing process. It needs to be consistently updated for it to be an effective method of symptom management.

So how do we go about assessing patient's physical symptoms? Again, there are a number of tools that you can use to do this. Links to many of these are available on the National End of Life Care Programme website (NEoLCP 2012a). One of the tools in common usage that may be useful in assessing physical symptoms is the Distress Thermometer (NEoLCP 2012b). The Distress Thermometer enables patients to rank the symptoms that are causing them the most distress using a visual analogue scale (VAS) in the form of a thermometer. It includes a list of symptoms, which reminds us and them of some of the common symptoms experienced by patients at the end of life.

When using the Distress Thermometer with Aarti, she identified that the main problems she had were: (1) breathing difficulties, (2) pain, (3) constipation, and (4) fatigue or exhaustion.

Keeping an ongoing record of the ranking scores of the different symptoms in Aarti's notes is useful. This allows us to assess what has been happening to her symptoms over time. The ranking scores provide a guide as to how to prioritise our symptom management. Aarti highlighted that her breathlessness was her most distressing symptom at present, so we need to start by looking at this. We need to assess each symptom carefully to explore the causative factors of the symptom so that we can target our management effectively. The following paragraphs will explore the assessment and management of some of the symptoms Aarti highlighted she was experiencing.

Assessing individual symptoms – breathlessness

Breathlessness or dyspnoea is the subjective experience of breathing discomfort (Campbell et al. 2010). Patients can be rated for this system in a number of ways, partially determined by their ability to participate in the assessment.

Aarti has identified that she struggles with shortness of breath. Behaviours may be another way to assess severity, particularly those related to functional ability. Aarti's breathlessness was impeding her mobility to the extent that she required a wheelchair to get from the car park to the clinic.

As with any symptom, investigation of the causative factors is very important so that appropriate interventions can be given. We are aware of Aarti's secondary (metastatic) disease in her lungs from her breast cancer. However, we also need to establish whether there may be any other more reversible factors that may be contributing to her symptoms.

Taking a history

Initially it is important to take a detailed history of the symptom. When someone is breathless, it may be most appropriate to involve the accompanying relative or to use a simple form for clarification with the patient, as history-giving when you are breathless can be very arduous.

This should include:

- information about onset – when, where and for how long;
- the nature of the breathlessness; and
- what exacerbates it and what relieves it.

Medications

It is important to look at what medications the patient is taking and when these were started or last changed to see if they relate to any development of symptoms.

Family history

Is there a history of respiratory problems in the family? Are there other underlying disease factors to consider?

Social history

A social history will include factors such as whether or not the patient is a smoker, whether he or she has dietary issues and whether there have been any recent stresses or exposures.

Examination

As nurses, we will do an initial physical examination, which will include observations of temperature, pulse rate, blood pressure, respiration rate, oxygen saturation on air, and perhaps a sputum sample if the patient has a productive cough. Medical or nurse practitioner colleagues will be able to conduct a more detailed physical examination and working collaboratively will give us even more information on which to base a possible diagnosis.

Ensuring that we start with a clear idea of the physiology of the respiratory process and then exploring the pathology (effect of disease) on our patient is essential in helping us think through what interventions are going to be helpful in this particular situation.

> ## Action point
>
> Select a patient you are looking after who has problems with breathlessness. Start by consulting a good nursing or medical textbook and explore the physiology of respiration. Look at your patient's notes and explore what factors may be influencing your patient's breathlessness. Perhaps with the help of one of the doctors on the ward, have a look at any X-rays or scans your patient has had of their chest area to give you as a full a picture of what is happening inside them and how this affects their normal breathing patterns.

Managing individual symptoms – breathlessness

To manage dyspnoea we need to return to the three tasks outlined by the *Palliative Care Toolkit* (Bond et al. 2008), starting with:

Task 1: Treat the treatable. With breathlessness, some reversible causes may include infection, which can be treated with antibiotics, corresponding cardiac impairment, which may require medication management, or some kind of thrombosis. It has already been established that our patient Aarti has metastatic disease in her lungs. If none of the above factors is evident, this may well be the cause of her breathlessness. She is already receiving treatment for her disease so this may need reviewing in light of her deterioration.

Task 2: Care for the patient. Gysels and Higginson (2011) undertook a study looking at the experience of breathlessness for patients with four different life-threatening illnesses. They found that the experience may be different for patients with different diagnoses, partly due to nature of the onset of the breathlessness, i.e. whether it was gradual or sudden, and partly due to the meaning that the patient may attribute to the feelings of the symptom.

For some patients, particularly those with cancer, breathlessness can be frightening and can be a signal of a severe deterioration in their health and also, perhaps, of their hopes. Exploring this with Aarti can be very supportive for a patient, particularly as feelings of anxiety can exacerbate feelings of breathlessness.

Bredin et al. (1999) did some useful work looking at the need for an integrated approach to be taken with people who are breathless. They recommend an approach that considers all the psychosocial factors as well as physical factors that will be contributing to this experience and have developed a behavioural model for dealing with long-term breathlessness.

Ensuring optimal positioning is important when some of the lung-expanding capacity may be compromised. Making sure your patient has a good supportive chair or position in bed where they can comfortably expand their chest cavity can help to reduce some feelings of breathlessness. Availability of fresh air to ensure a flow of air either through the use of doors and windows or by using a fan may also improve the feeling of breathlessness. Breathlessness can cause and be exacerbated by stress so complementary therapies such as reflexology, acupuncture and some simple massage or aromatherapy can be very helpful for patients as part of a longer-term management plan. However, Brennan and Mazanec (2011) remind us that there is research work to be done to validate these strategies.

Task 3: Using palliative care drugs. When working with all patients with dyspnoea, care needs to be taken before offering piped oxygen as a way of managing this symptom in patients with long-term and non-reversible causes. A dependency on oxygen can result in the complication of providing this support at home and is not always beneficial in the long term. There are other measures that can be employed to help reduce often frightening feelings of running out of breath.

Once the causal factors have been established, appropriate treatments can be offered. Understanding the use of medications in the management of breathlessness is a good place to start. In some cases, such as patients with COPD, it may be a symptom that the patient has had to manage for some time. The patient may already be on medication, such as bronchodilators, to manage this. They are often used in combination and dose increases may be appropriate as the patient's airway capacity decreases. The National Institute for Clinical Evidence (NICE) guidelines for COPD (NICE 2010) offer an evidence-based discussion of these medications and their role in the management of this disease, and Yohannes (2007) offers a helpful explanation about how these may work for the patient. They both also look at psychosocial interventions and pulmonary rehabilitation.

The use of morphine, using either the oral or parental route (it is also given using the nebulised route but there is limited evidence of its effectiveness) can be particularly beneficial in patients with breathlessness at the end of life (Brennan and Mazanec 2011). The use of a low dose of morphine can help to reduce the sensation of breathlessness. Sometimes it is also useful to add in a benzodiazepine.

Reflective questions

Sitting with a patient like Aarti, who is having difficulty breathing, can be a frightening and distressing experience for anyone. It often makes us feel increasingly anxious and we start to panic too. Aarti has been started on some low dose oral morphine and some bronchodilators. She is aware that this deterioration is an indication that her disease is progressing and she has an appointment to see the consultant in clinic later in the week.

Think about how you might be able to care for Aarti and prepare her for going home. How would you maintain a calm approach? Using Bredin et al.'s integrated model (1999), how would you use a behavioural approach to help her and her daughter think about how they may help Aarti to feel more comfortable?

Ongoing assessment and evaluation

Brennan and Mazanec (2011) discuss the usefulness of the Medical Research Council (MRC) dyspnoea scale assessment in end-of-life care as it measures the extent to which breathlessness impairs mobility and functioning. This can be used with the patient to look at a baseline point and then be used to monitor changes in their breathlessness as they go along. They emphasise the importance of regular and ongoing assessment, particularly using self-report mechanisms, in providing an accurate picture of this complex symptom.

Grade degree of breathlessness related to activities

1 Not troubled by breathlessness except on strenuous exercise.
2 Short of breath when hurrying or walking up a slight hill.
3 Walks slower than contemporaries on level ground because of breathlessness or has to stop for breath when walking at own pace.
4 Stops for breath after walking about 100 metres or after a few minutes on level ground.
5 Too breathless to leave the house or breathless when dressing or undressing. (NICE 2007)

Assessing individual symptoms – pain

Why do we experience pain? Cicely Saunders (1978), the founder of the modern hospice movement, described a concept known as 'total pain'. She explored how the pain of terminal disease is a combination of social, spiritual and psychological factors which together affect the physical experience of pain. Many of the factors that cause this total pain have already been explored earlier in the book. This section will concentrate on the management of physical pain. Physical pain is a complex symptom and requires good decision-making to achieve the best outcomes.

Knowledge is a key player in good decision-making. It is useful to be aware of the different types of pain and the way that pain pathways work to help with decision-making about pain management (Paz and Seymour 2008). There is a large amount of literature available about pain and a number of different theories which try to understand why we experience different sensations of pain. Melzack and Wall (1996) developed an interesting neurological gate control theory which is helpful in understanding why heat pads and rubbing of an area may help to relieve pain. This is nicely summarised in an article by Ngugi (2007) which may be worth reading to enhance your understanding of the sensation of pain.

Types of pain

Briggs (2010a) discusses three types of pain: (1) acute pain, which she sees as the pain that occurs as a warning sign to indicate damage or injury; (2) chronic or persistent pain; and (3) cancer pain, which she describes as pain associated with malignancy. She offers this third type of pain because it denotes the often multifactorial nature of the pain in cancer.

Pain can be caused by the effect of the tumour on surrounding structures as well as from the treatments for cancer. Treatments can weaken body systems, resulting in patients being more prone to pain such as skin damage, muscle damage, etc. Pain of any type has a variety of origins and for the purposes of this book we will look at nociceptive pain, neuropathic pain, bone pain and cancer pain.

Nociceptive pain

Nociceptors are receptors that sense when there is tissue injury or damage. They pick up changes in the chemical, thermal or mechanical environment in the tissues (Briggs 2010b) that are a result of the injury and the body's inflammatory response to that injury. This response includes the release of prostaglandins, serotonin, histamine, bradykinin and substance P. The chemicals produced by the inflammatory response and injury stimulate the sensory nerve endings (Paice 2004) and the information is converted into electrical impulses that carry the messages to the brain via the nervous system.

Neuropathic pain

Neuropathic pain refers to pain that occurs as a result of neurological damage. Symptoms of neuropathic pain include sensations of stabbing, tingling, perhaps pins and needles, burning and shooting pains. It can also result in hypersensitisation of areas of the skin or allodynia, where even a slight touch or brush against something can cause an intensely painful feeling.

Neurological pain can be as a result of peripheral nerve involvement or central nerve involvement so can be complex to diagnose and to treat. However, it is useful if we can identify the different types of pain our patient may have as we may need a combination of management strategies to achieve the best outcomes for them.

Bone pain and cancer pain

This term 'cancer pain' covers a number of different elements, although one of the most common and more unique types of pain that we see in cancer management is that of metastatic bone pain. This can be a combination of nociceptive pain and neurological pain. The most common physiology for this type of pain is destruction of bone tissue as a result of disease and tumour growth that can press on nerve endings. This is ideally managed by treating the disease, or halting or slowing down the metastatic process in the bone through a combination of anti-cancer therapies such as chemotherapy and radiotherapy, but also through the use of bisphosphonates which strengthen bone tissue. However, if you are unable to treat the disease, bone pain can be challenging to manage.

Using analgesia

Understanding the origins of pain and the pain pathways involved can help us think about what analgesia we may want to use and why it is often helpful to use more than one type.

NSAIDS (non-steroidal anti-inflammatory drugs) and corticosteroids such as dexamethasone block the formation of prostaglandins in the tissues so are useful medications in the control of pain that initiates in the tissues, i.e. nociceptive pain.

Opioids, such as morphine, relieve pain primarily by binding with opioid receptors in the spinal cord which inhibit the release of neurotransmitters in the dorsal horns (Paice 2004) and so reduce the number of pain signals that get past this point. For this reason, opioids are useful analgesics for a wide range of situations.

One of the systems discussed by Melzack and Wall (1996) that can be used to help control pain is the idea that some neurological messages that are being sent back down the system, from the brain back to the tissues. This is sometimes called descending systems. These neurological impulses originate in structures deep in the middle of the brain or what is called the brain stem. These descending messages cause the release of neurotransmitters such as serotonin and noradrenaline (known as norepinephrine in the USA) (Paice 2004). These substances are thought to enhance mood and perhaps lessen the effect of the pain stimuli. Tricyclic antidepressants such as amitriptyline block the re-uptake of these substances so when you administer these drugs, the neurotransmitters remain in greater volumes than normal and offer a reducing effect on pain, particularly neuropathic pain. It is important to note that the effect of tricyclic antidepressants is not immediate, as with other analgesia, but the effect builds up over a matter of days to weeks.

Other pathways that appear to modulate the expression of neuropathic pain include the GABA neurotransmitter pathways. Exactly how this works is complex and under debate. However, gabapentin is a drug whose molecules appear very similar to that of the neurotransmitter GABA so it acts to enhance the modulating effect of this pathway.

Managing individual symptoms – pain

Task 1: Treat the treatable. Aarti is currently having a course of chemotherapy which is aiming to treat the underlying cause of her symptoms, which is her cancer. Careful review is required of patients on treatment who continue to develop symptoms to ensure that the treatment is remaining effective. Ensuring Aarti and her daughter feel confident about discussing her symptoms with the medical staff when she is being reviewed is an important part of her care.

Task 2: Care for the patient. It is important to have a clear idea of the type of pain Aarti is experiencing and the effect it is having on her life in order to offer person-centred care. Aarti had ranked pain as her second most distressing physical symptom on her Distress Thermometer scale. It will be useful to get a full history of the symptom. In this example we are assessing each symptom separately. In reality, some of the questions we ask in our general assessment will feed into each symptom exploration, for example previous medical history, family and social history, medications and physical appearance. The *Gold Standards Toolkit* (Gold Standards Framework 2012) offers the SCR5 pain assessment chart where this type of information can be recorded for use by all the team (see Figure 6.1).

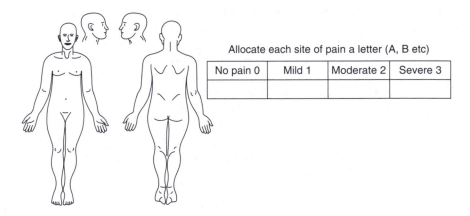

Allocate each site of pain a letter (A, B etc)

No pain 0	Mild 1	Moderate 2	Severe 3

Figure 6.1   Pain assessment chart (Gold Standards Framework 2012)

With any symptom, one of the simplest and most well-used tool is the PQRST pneumonic which allows you to explore the patient's experience of the symptom. This was originally developed to encourage culturally competent chest pain assessment (Kernicki 1993) although it can be used in a variety of situations.

P – Provokes/precipitating factors. What starts the pain or where does it feel it is coming from? What makes it feel better or feel worse (e.g. movement)? It may be helpful to assess this element using a body outline and asking the patient to indicate on the chart the different areas of pain they are experiencing. You can then number these pains and work with them separately as they may be different types of pain and so respond to different types of management.

Q – Quality of pain. What does it feel like? Intermittent or constant? How would you describe it?

R – Region and radiation. Does it stay in one place, move or radiate from its origin? This often gives us an indication of whether there is neuropathic pain involved.

S – Severity or associated symptoms. On a score of 1–10, how would you rate your pain right now, today, this week? A number of what are known as visual analogue scales (VAS) are available for this. These allows the patient to indicate where on the scale they rate their pain.

T – Temporal factors/timing. When did you first feel this pain? When does it come on – any particular part of the day, week or year?

(Adapted from Briggs 2010a)

Reflective questions

Explore the pain chart at your place of work. Which of these elements does it contain?

What other areas are on the chart?

Where a patient's pain is complex and perhaps likely to require ongoing management, it may be appropriate to explore it using one of the more complex pain tools such as the adapted McGill Pain Questionnaire (Wright et al. 2001).

The following is an outline of the pain assessment carried out on Aarti.

Provokes/precipitating factors. Aarti reported that she has two main areas of pain, in her mid-spine and in her upper left arm. Her pain is always present but it feels worse on movement and by the end of the day. She is on some regular pain medication and has tried using hot water bottles. She also has a number of special pillows that she uses in bed. She has found herself minimising movement to prevent the pain but as a result has had trouble with her bowels. This in turn put her off taking too many pain killers.

Quality of pain. She describes the pain as a throbbing pain that becomes more intense when putting pressure on her arm or back or moving them. Her back pain is more intense more of the time.

Region and radiation. She feels the pain is fairly fixed to the areas, although sometimes on movement she does get a shooting pain down her back.

Severity or associated symptoms. She scored the pains as a 5 for her arm pain and a 7–8 for her back pain. She feels that it doesn't vary too much from this most of the time.

Temporal factors/timing. She is finding it difficult to sleep as she finds it painful to change position and reposition herself. She also wakes during the night and has to take pain killers.

Task 3: Using palliative care drugs. The World Health Organisation has developed three principles that are useful to consider when using palliative care drugs to manage pain.

Principle 1: By the mouth. Where possible, the oral route should always be used. Try and avoid intramuscular or intravenous routes unless specifically indicated.

Principle 2: By the clock. Analgesia should be given at regular intervals to prevent the pain from coming back, rather than waiting for the pain to remerge. Higher doses of medication will be required to control pain that is established rather than pain that is being kept at bay by regular medication. PRN (as required) medications should be reserved for breakthrough doses of analgesia or if the pain is intermittent.

Principle 3: By the ladder. This refers to the three-step WHO analgesic ladder. The ladder approach suggests the use of a slowly up-scaling response involving opioids medications for increasing pain management and a similarly step fashion of decreasing pain management when the cause of the pain is alleviating. The analgesic ladder was first developed for the control of cancer pain in the 1980s. It has been widely used to legitimate the use of morphine as a major player in pain control and to try to prevent inadequate pain relief from being given.

 The ladder suggests that you start with non-opioid analgesic medications such as aspirin or paracetamol, ensuring you are using the drug to its maximum dose and the patient is receiving it regularly. Adjuvant drugs are other types of medication that may also offer pain relief by working on different pathways or through different mechanisms. These include the non-steroidal anti-inflammatories and medications like steroids that can also have an anti-inflammatory effect.

If the patient is still in pain, the ladder proposes that you may continue to use a non-opioid like paracetamol but may add in a mild opioid such as the codeine-based range of medications or tramadol. If any of these medications contain paracetamol, additional paracetamol must not be used as taking more than the recommended 4g in 24 hours can be harmful. Again, with this level, care needs to be taken to ensure regular and appropriate dosing.

If your patient continues to experience pain, having first established the types of pain they may be experiencing and ensuring you have tried appropriate adjuvant medications for neurological or bone pain, it may be appropriate to move to the strong opioid medications which include the morphine-based medications, oxycodone and fentanyl. (See Figure 6.2.)

Since its early development, the analgesic ladder has been revaluated and adapted to cover other conditions. Vargas-Schaffer (2010) has produced the updated ladder for use with cancer and non-malignant pain. It recognises there are still situations

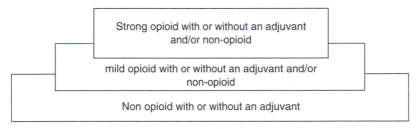

Figure 6.2 The three-step analgesic ladder (adapted from WHO 2012)

where it may not be appropriate, such as severe sudden onset pain where a stepwise approach may need to be avoided. The WHO is currently working on new guidelines which look separately at acute pain, chronic cancer pain and chronic non-malignant pain.

Returning to our patient Aarti, it is important to look at what types of medications she is currently on. Aarti has been prescribed co-dydramol. She has tended only to take a few tablets each day as it caused constipation. She was also taking paracetamol in the night, which she has done for some time, and some ibuprofen if the pain got very bad. Patients don't always realise the paracetamol content in medications such as co-dydramol and risk overdosing with the mild opioid medications.

For Aarti, who is currently on the second step of the ladder and still experiencing significant pain, it would be appropriate to raise her to the third step of the ladder. Patients who have not had morphine-based medications may sometimes find this a difficult step. There are some commonly held misconceptions about the use of morphine, sometimes referred to as the 'morphine myths', which associate the prescription of morphine with impending death. Stannard (2008) explores some of these anxieties. It may be useful to review these in preparation for questions you may be asked by patients or families. It may also be useful to remind people of the now common use of morphine in post-operative pain management with PCAs (patient-controlled analgesia pumps).

For many patients starting on a morphine-based regime, they may initially experience side-effects of drowsiness, or a 'spaced out' feeling, dry mouth or some nausea. It is important to warn patients and families of these effects, assess frequently, and offer appropriate antiemetics if required. These initial side-effects often wear off if the dosage is correct. Morphine slows down the activity of smooth muscle so it will cause the bowel to slow down and a very common side-effect is constipation. It is therefore important to ensure a regular aperient is prescribed and then your patient's bowel movements are regularly assessed.

Due to the nature of bone pain and its severity, you might also maintain Aarti's regular non-steroidal anti-inflammatory. You would need to discuss these medications with Aarti and her daughter carefully and clarify their understanding of the rationale behind this medication change.

Assessing individual symptoms – constipation and diarrhoea

Bowel care is a complex issue for many patients, partly due to issues of dignity and disclosure. However, constipation is a common symptom that can result in extreme suffering. It can also cause an increase in other symptoms, such as pain due to a reluctance to take medication that may result in worsening constipation. If unresolved, constipation can become very serious and lead to bowel obstruction.

The aim of symptom control in this area is initially to relieve discomfort but it is also primarily to help the patient to return to a normal elimination pattern. A group of clinicians in palliative care, mainly nurses and doctors, have compiled some useful guidelines for good practice (Larkin et al. 2008).

Managing individual symptoms – constipation and diarrhoea

Returning to our principles of treating the treatable, it is important to assess the situation carefully, taking into account the many factors that may influence the bowel patterns. For the patient at the end of life, there are usually a number of different factors leading to the experience of constipation. Movement will often be restricted, and a lack of movement can have a depressive effect on bowel peristalsis. Appetite and fluid consumption may have changed, and this may result in a reduction of movement through the bowel, which slows down the rate of food passing through, and a reduction in foods high in fibre and liquids that increase the rate of food passage through the gastrointestinal (GI) system. There may also be direct effects from the disease or illness the person has, such as tumours or reduced muscle and nervous control. Almost inevitably they will be on a number of medications which cause a reduced bowel peristalsis as a side-effect.

Aarti has already been troubled by constipation and this had made her reluctant to take her full dose of analgesia. It is always extremely important that patients are started on some type of laxative/aperient when they start taking codeine- or morphine-based medication, particularly when their mobility and probably their diet are also affected. Many patients may require both a softener, which will increase the absorption of fluid into the bowel and make faecal matter easier to pass, and a stimulant, which will encourage peristalsis. Some medications can offer an element of both of these actions. Advising regular doses to start with until a normal bowel pattern is established should make Aarti feel much better.

Assessing individual symptoms – fatigue or tiredness

At end of life, one of the more frequently cited symptoms suffered by patients with a variety of conditions is fatigue (Solano et al. 2006). Fatigue associated with advanced disease is described as an excessive sense of tiredness that is not relieved through rest. Many patients find that fatigue results in severely impairing their lives as they become debilitatingly tired after only a short time or undertaking even simple regular action such as having a bath. However although it is widely experienced, patients don't always consider it a symptom to be reported like pain or perhaps nausea, as there is almost a sense of inevitability about it. This is perhaps exacerbated by professionals who often offer false assurances to patients raising their problems with fatigue with responses such as … 'oh don't worry, you will soon feel better,' or 'you just need a good rest'. Families can also hinder by pressuring patients to eat high calorie diets thinking this will replenish energy stores and so alleviate the problem.

The European Association for Palliative Care (EAPC et al. 2008) have developed a position paper on the management of fatigue in palliative care which offers some helpful information, particularly around the definition of fatigue. The discussion helps to highlight the complex nature of this symptom and also the limited assessment and management that occurs. They suggest that all patients with palliative care needs should be screened with a question such as 'Do you feel unusually tired or weak?' If the response is positive, further assessment should be undertaken.

As a result of this wide variety of definition, there has been a significant number of assessment tools developed (Whitehead 2009). The Fatigue Severity Scale (FSS) developed by Krupp et al. in 1989, is one of the best known and most widely used tools and has been used successfully with a number of patients with different conditions. Our patient, Aarti, has identified fatigue and exhaustion as a major problem for her. It may be useful to explore this further using the FSS.

The Fatigue Severity Scale (FSS)

The FSS questionnaire contains nine statements about the manner in which fatigue affects the patient. This tool involves asking the patient, using a visual analogue scale (VAS), to rate the severity of fatigue symptoms.

When asked, Aarti, using a VAS scoring between 0 and 7 found that over the past week she had:

	Score
1 My motivation is lower when I am fatigued.	5
2 Exercise brings on my fatigue.	7
3 I am easily fatigued.	7
4 Fatigue interferes with my physical functioning.	6
5 Fatigue causes frequent problems for me.	6
6 My fatigue prevents sustained physical functioning.	5
7 Fatigue interferes with carrying out certain duties and responsibilities.	7
8 Fatigue is among my three most disabling symptoms.	6
9 Fatigue interferes with my work, family, or social life.	5

(Krupp et al. 1989).

The scoring is done by adding up all the answers and dividing by nine and getting a mean score. In Krupp et al.'s original study (1989), they found that the control sample of normal healthy adults has mean scores of around 2.3. However, their sample of patients with multiple sclerosis (MS) scored mean scores around 4.8 and patients with systemic lupus erthromytosis (SLE) scored around 4.7.

For Aarti this is a score of 6 which gives us some indication of how severe this problem is for her.

The tool itself does not give guidelines as to when a score is significant, but with a base line of normal healthy adults at 2.3, scores significantly higher than this indicate the severity of the patient's symptom. This scale also allows for a longitudinal assessment of the patient's symptom to be made and to look at their experience of the symptom over time.

Because of the subjective nature of fatigue as a symptom, the EAPC recommend that assessment of fatigue should depend on self-evaluation by the patient. This should only be substituted by estimations of carers or staff where self-assessment is not possible (EAPC et al. 2008).

Managing individual symptoms – fatigue

Fatigue remains a complex symptom to manage effectively so a guiding priority has to be remembering that people often have very little energy left to care for themselves and achieve the things that are important to them. Helping someone to complete the basic care requirements of hygiene, nutrition and elimination can preserve valuable energy, as well as enable them to feel more able to look forward and make plans. Alternatively suggesting that they perhaps wash at night rather than in the morning can enable them to use their morning energy to complete a task or outing they want to do, which perhaps would feel too overwhelming after exhausting themselves having a bath or shower.

Management plans involve firstly acknowledging the symptom and assessing it like you would other symptoms and then helping patients to set small achievable goals and by exploring their energy patterns and prioritising actions to enable them to do the things they want to do most.

The EAPC (2008) paper also concludes that in the final stage of life, fatigue may provide protection, shielding the patient from suffering, and thus treatment of this symptom may be detrimental. Identification of the point of time where the treatment of fatigue is no longer indicated is important to alleviate distress at the end of life.

Other difficult symptoms

Corner (2008) offers a useful consideration of some of the more challenging and often unnoticed symptoms that patients experience at the end of life, such as odour and exudates, which are important considerations if our aim of care is to promote well-being.

Action point

Explore the symptoms that are most commonly described by your patients and investigate their pathophysiology and management. What are the more hidden symptoms or less common symptoms that perhaps challenge the health care team you work with?

Think about asking for this to be put on the ward or class agenda for discussion and perhaps some teaching.

In conclusion, and returning to our initial symptom assessment of Aarti, we can see that many of her symptoms are deteriorating, indicating a progression of disease despite the chemotherapy she is receiving. Her feeling of well-being is also deteriorating, so it may well indicate the need to review her current treatment plan and to discuss with Aarti and her daughter what the next move should be. This type of communication is important in achieving good outcomes in end-of-life care for our patients. However, it is challenging and can lead to difficult and upsetting conversations. Chapter 3 looks at some of these aspects of communication and offers some strategies for planning for and managing these types of conversation.

Summary

The key points to remember when managing a patient's symptoms are:

- It is important to conduct a clear assessment of the symptoms of your patient.
- Use the three principles of management: treat the treatable, care for the patient and use palliative care drugs.
- Understanding the underlying physiology of the symptom and the treatments enables you to offer more specific interventions.
- Consider both pharmacological and non-pharmacological interventions.
- Regular reassessment and evaluation is important in achieving successful long-term effectiveness.

Further reading

Chapter 5 of Bond, C., Wooldrige, R. and Lavy, V. (2008) *The Palliative Care Toolkit*. London: Help the Hospices, offers a useful exploration of pain management and reminds us of some of the basic important principles we need to apply to pain management. Use this resource to critically explore:

- Managing somatic pain. This requires a good understanding of different types of opioid medications, their different characteristics and dosage ranges, including the use of the World Health Organisation's 'pain ladder'.
- Types of adjuvant medications commonly used in end-of-life care.
- Managing other types of pain – inflammatory pain, nerve pain, muscle spasm and abdominal cramps.

Watson, M., Lucas, C., Hoy, A. and Wells, J. (2009) *The Oxford Textbook of Palliative Care*. Oxford: Oxford Medical Publications, is a useful book for managing more complex symptoms.

Chapter 8 of Nyatanga, B. (2008) *Why Is It So Difficult to Die?* (2nd edn). London: Quay Books, explores some ways to help us to understand our patients' experience better. This helps us to provide a more holistic approach, particularly to the phenomenon of total pain.

References

Bond, C., Wooldrige, R. and Lavy, V. (2008) *The Palliative Care Toolkit*. London: Help the Hospices.

Bredin, M., Corner, J., Krishnasamy, M., Plant, H., Bailey, C. and A'Hern, R. (1999) 'Multicentre RCT of nursing intervention for breathlessness in patients with lung cancer', *British Medical Journal*, 318: 901–4.

Brennan, C.W. and Mazanec, P. (2011) 'Dyspnea management across the palliative care continuum', *Journal of Hospice & Palliative Nursing*, 13(3): 130–9.

Briggs, E. (2010a) 'Assessment and expression of pain', *Nursing Standard*, 25(2): 35–8.

Briggs, E. (2010b) 'Understanding the experience and physiology of pain', *Nursing Standard*, 25(3): 35–9.

Burt, J., Shipman, C., Richardson, A., Ream, E. and Addington-Hall, J. (2010) 'The experiences of older adults in the community dying from cancer and non-cancer causes: a national survey of bereaved relatives', *Age and Ageing*, 39(1): 86–91.

Campbell, M., Templin, T. and Walch, J. (2010) 'A respiratory distress observation scale for patients unable to self-report dyspnoea', *Journal of Palliative Medicine*, 13(3): 285–90.

Corner, J. (2008) 'Working with difficult symptoms', Chapter 12 in S. Payne, J. Seymour and C. Ingleton (eds), *Palliative Care Nursing: Principles and Evidence for Practice* (2nd edn). Buckingham: Open University Press.

Dittner, A., Wessely, S. and Brown, R. (2004) 'The assessment of fatigue: a practical guide for clinicians and researchers', *Journal of Psychosomatic Research*, 56: 157–70.

EAPC (Research Steering Committee of the European Association for Palliative Care), Radbruch, L., Strasser, F., Elsner, F., Ferraz Gonçalves, J., Løge, J., Kaasa, S., Nauck, F. and Stone, P. (2008) 'Fatigue in palliative care patients: an EAPC approach', *Palliative Medicine*, 22(1): 13–22.

Gold Standards Framework (2012) *Gold Standards Toolkit* [online]. Available at: www.goldstandardsframework.org.uk/TheGSFToolkit [accessed 25 May 2012].

Gysels, M.H. and Higginson, I.J. (2011) 'The lived experience of breathlessness and its implications for care: a qualitative comparison in cancer, COPD, heart failure and MND', *BMC Palliative Care*, (10): 15. Available at: www.biomedcentral.com/1472-684X/10/15 [accessed 25 May 2012]

Kernicki, J. (1993) 'Differentiating chest pain: advanced assessment techniques', *Dimensions of Critical Care Nursing*, 12: 66–76.

Krupp, L.B., LaRocca, N.G., Muir-Nash, J. and Steinberg, A.D. (1989) 'The fatigue severity scale: application to patients with multiple sclerosis and systemic lupus erythematosus', *Archives of Neurology*, 46: 1121–3.

Larkin, P.J., Sykes, N. et al. (2008) 'The management of constipation in palliative care: clinical practice recommendations', *Palliative Medicine*, 22: 796–807.

Melzack, R. and Wall, P.D. (1996) *The Challenge of Pain* (2nd edn). Harmondsworth: Penguin.

National End of Life Care Programme (NEoLCP) (2012a) [online]. Available at: www.endoflifecareforadults.nhs.uk/ [accessed 25 May 2012)].

National End of Life Care Programme (NEoLCP) (2012b) *Distress Thermometer* [online]. Available at: www.endoflifecareforadults.nhs.uk/tools/emerging-practice/needs-assessment-pathway/tools-and-documents/distress-thermometer [accessed 25 May 2012].

Ngugi, V. (2007) 'Managing neuropathic pain in end-stage carcinoma', *End of Life Care*, 1(1): 38–46.

NICE (National Institute for Health and Clinical Excellence) (2007) *MRC Dyspnoea Scale*. Available online at: www.nice.org.uk/usingguidance/commissioningguides/pulmonaryrehabilitationserviceforpatientswithcopd/mrc_dyspnoea_scale.jsp [accessed 11 September 2012].

NICE (2010) *Chronic Obstructive Pulmonary Disease* (updated) (CG101) [online]. Available at: http://guidance.nice.org.uk/CG101 [accessed 11 September 2012].

Paice, J. (2004) 'Pain', Chapter 9 in C. Yarbro, M. Hansen and M. Goodman (eds), *Cancer Symptom Management* (3rd edn). Jones and Bartlett Series in Oncology. USA: Jones and Bartlett Publishers.

Paz, S. and Seymour, J. (2008) 'Pain: theories, evaluation and management', in S. Payne, J. Seymour and C. Ingleton (eds), *Palliative Care Nursing: Principles and Evidence for Practice* (2nd edn). Buckingham: Open University Press.

Saunders, C. (1978) 'The philosophy of terminal care', in C. Saunders (ed.), *The Management of Terminal Disease*. London: Edward Arnold.

Solano, J.P., Gomes, B. and Higginson, I.J. (2006) 'A comparison of symptom prevalence in far advanced cancer, AIDS, heart disease, chronic obstructive pulmonary disease and renal disease', *Journal Pain and Symptom Management*, 31(1): 58–69.

Stannard, S. (2008) 'Morphine: dispelling the myths and the misconceptions', *End of Life Care Journal*, 2(3): 7–12.

Vargas-Schaffer, G. (2010) 'Is the WHO analgesic ladder still valid? Twenty-four years of experience', *Canadian Family Physician*, 56(6): 514–17.

Whitehead, L. (2009) 'The measurement of fatigue in chronic illness: a systematic review of uni-dimensional and multidimensional fatigue measures', *Journal of Pain and Symptom Management*, 37(1): 107.

WHO (2012) World Health Organization Definition of Palliative Care [online]. Available at: www.who.int/cancer/palliative/definition/en/ [accessed 11 September 2012].

Wright, K., Asmundson, G. and McCreary, D. (2001) 'Factorial validity of the short-form McGill pain questionnaire (SF-MPQ)', *European Journal of Pain*, 5(3): 279–84.

Yohannes, A. (2007) 'Palliative care provision for patients with chronic obstructive pulmonary disease', *Health and Quality of Life Outcomes*, 5: 17.

CHAPTER 7

Discharging patients approaching the end of life

Annie Pettifer

This chapter will explore:

- Supporting patients going home from hospital
- Supporting someone who doesn't feel able to cope with their dying relative at home
- Planning the care of someone whose needs are changing
- The services available to people who need end-of-life care at home
- Co-ordinating discharge planning
- Co-ordinating end-of-life care in the community

Introduction

Planning the discharge of patients from hospital to their homes is a key role of nurses and health care practitioners (Lees 2007). Although ward-based nurses may not see the results of careful discharge planning, it is crucial to the care of people facing the end of their lives who wish to be in their own homes.

This chapter opens with a case study involving a student caring for a person whose health is rapidly deteriorating and who wants to go home. The chapter explores the difficulties of planning discharge to home of patients who are very unwell, and the organisation of end-of-life care services in the community. The nature and funding of community services will be detailed, together with principles of referring to them. Once again, while one case is followed, the principles of care involved are extractable to the care of many.

Mr Sevim

Helen is a third-year student nurse on her management placement on an oncology ward. One Thursday afternoon, she was asked by her mentor to accompany Dr Hughes, a medical oncologist, on his ward round. She was to act as a nursing resource and conduit for any decisions made by the medical team. During the round, the team saw Ahmed Sevim, a 68 year-old Turkish shopkeeper.

Mr Sevim first presented to his GP 15 months ago complaining of an irritating cough, weight loss and fatigue. Following a suspicious chest X-ray result, he was referred to a chest physician who diagnosed non-small cell adenocarcinoma of the lung on bronchoscopy. Staging investigation revealed staging of 3a, the cancer having infiltrated into the mediastinal lymph nodes in his chest. Unfortunately the tumour was not suitable for surgical resection and Mr Sevim received radiotherapy followed by chemotherapy. For some months following this, his symptoms improved. However, over the last two months he has been feeling more and more unwell. He presented at clinic complaining of increasing fatigue, weakness, weight loss and pain, both in his chest and right hip. Further investigations showed his tumour had spread both within his chest and to a number of sites in his bones. His pain was treated with a single fraction of radiotherapy to his hip and with oral morphine. Although his symptoms have been well controlled, during his 10-day admission he has clearly become weaker.

On the ward round, Dr Hughes confirmed Mr Sevim's suspicion that his disease had advanced extensively and that he would not benefit from further radiotherapy or chemotherapy to alleviate his disease. When asked, Dr Hughes confirmed Mr Sevim's suspicions that he was likely to die in the next few weeks.

Mr Sevim said he would prefer to go home to spend his remaining life with his wife and family. Looking directly at Helen, Dr Hughes told Mr Sevim that discharge home, with some help to care for him there, would be planned as soon as possible.

Early in the evening, Helen sat down with Mr Sevim to discuss what Dr Hughes had said and to assess Mr Sevim's care needs at home. Fortunately, Mrs Sevim arrived for her evening visit and the three could make plans together. Helen's assessment found that they were keen for discharge to home quickly as they realised that Mr Sevim's condition was deteriorating rapidly. Currently, he needs the help of at least one person to move from his bed to a chair as he is weak and breathless much of the time. His pain is currently stable and is controlled by oral morphine, but it is likely to exacerbate in the future. He is experiencing a small amount of haemoptysis (coughing up blood). Going home is clearly imperative to Mr Sevim. However, although Mrs Sevim seems supportive of her husband's wish, she is more tentative about the discharge and says repeatedly that she does not want to be involved in her husband's personal care. She emphasises her role of shopping and cooking, and is anxious that she may be unable to cope with more, both practically and emotionally. She is partially-sighted but otherwise reasonably well. They live in a three-bedroom house that unfortunately has no downstairs toilet. They have helpful neighbours but no local family.

Helen left the couple with a clear but daunting picture of their circumstances. She wonders if sufficient services at home can be arranged quickly enough given the debility and limited prognosis, and particularly when Mrs Sevim can offer only limited practical support and is clearly anxious. She wonders whether perhaps discharge to home is the right decision.

Sometimes, faced with the news of rapidly advancing disease and, in all likelihood, death in a few days or weeks, patients will wish to go home and spend the remaining time with their families in familiar surroundings. However, the provision of services to meet the complex and changing needs of dying patients at home, often at short notice, can be difficult or even impossible. The length of time it takes to assess and arrange services can be frustrating and sometimes, sadly, patients die in hospital while waiting for services at home to be ready. It is also common to be concerned about a patient discharged home to services that may prove inadequate to meet their needs. Sometimes, if this is the case, patients may go home only to return to hospital a few days later.

These challenges are real and shared by many health care professionals. However, there are a number of strategies that can be used to minimise them, and to enable patients to be discharged home should they wish.

Supporting patients going home from hospital

The support of dying patients and their families when they are in the process of considering where to spend their remaining life demands great sensitivity. Commonly, patients come into hospital when they are sick, and are discharged when they are considerably better and are more capable of caring for themselves at home. Given this norm, it is not surprising that discharging patients who are approaching the end of their lives, and who are in fact considerably more sick at the time of discharge than when they were when admitted to hospital, is daunting. It can be tempting to feel, as Helen does, that in fact they are too unwell to be cared for adequately at home, and therefore must be cared for in hospital. However, when patients like Mr Sevim cannot benefit from the diagnostic care and treatment available within hospital, end-of-life care can be provided in a number of other settings. Consequently, there is a choice to be made, and it is imperative that we are clear as to who should make that choice and how.

> ## Reflective questions
>
> You may recollect key principles about decision-making from Chapter 4. Relate the key principles of the Mental Capacity Act 2005 to Mr Sevim's situation and consider the following questions:
>
> - Who should decide whether or not Mr Sevim can go home?
> - What is the appropriate role of Helen in caring for Mr Sevim?

The principles set out in the Mental Capacity Act 2005 (UK Parliament, 2005) and explained in the Mental Capacity Act 2005 Code of Practice 2007 (Department of Constitutional Affairs 2007) make it clear that every adult has the right to make his or her own decisions, and must be assumed to have capacity to do so unless it is established otherwise (Department of Constitutional Affairs 2007). Therefore, in this case, decisions regarding Mr Sevim's health care lie with him. While Helen's apprehensions are reasonable, she must respect his wishes. Research tells us that being cared for and dying within your own home is important for many people (Townsend et al. 1990; Higginson and Sen-Gupta 2000; Higginson 2003). The UK government aims to ensure that quality care at the end of life is available to all, regardless of their choice of place (Department of Health 2008). Whether this choice is met is increasingly used as an indicator of the quality of care patients receive (Munday et el. 2007).

Although Mr Sevim has strong views about where he is to be cared for, other patients may prefer a family member to make decisions on their behalf or simply to adopt the choice recommended by professionals. All of these options are valid and should be respected.

Helen's role in the decision-making process is firstly to provide realistic advice about what care and support is available to Mr and Mrs Sevim at home. It may take time to establish this. Helen should be very careful not to promise services that are not in fact available. Sometimes patients may hold unrealistic expectations such as having two nurses present in the home continually, or remaining in hospital indefinitely. It may be helpful to give information about realistic alternatives such as discharge to a hospice once a bed is available.

Once it is clear what care can be offered to Mr and Mrs Sevim at home, Helen's role is to help Mr Sevim weigh up the information and make a choice. It may be helpful to explore his hopes and expectations about life at home, and advise whether or not these are realistic. At this point it may be important to state what risks might be involved. For example, it may take longer to provide additional pain control if Mr Sevim unexpectedly and urgently requires it. Be aware that patients do change their minds, particularly as their health gets worse and leaving hospital may become more daunting.

Once patients have clear information about the choices available to them, their wishes can be documented as part of advance care planning. Given the strength of

Mr Sevim's desire to go home, it is likely that he would welcome the opportunity to document this. Health care organisations may have differing systems for documenting patients' care preferences. One example of this is the Preferred Priorities for Care document (PPC) (see Further reading for website address). Lancaster and South Cumbria Cancer Network originally devised this as a patient-held record of the preferred place of care for people approaching the end of their lives at home. It was strongly endorsed by the National End of Life Care Programme in 2007, and broadened to enable recording of general patient care preferences as the end of life approaches. PPC documents are considered as 'advance decisions' if patients lose capacity and decisions have to be made in their best interest (as discussed in Chapter 4). The PPC record can travel with Mr Sevim to ensure that the integrated care team caring for him at home are clear about his preferences.

Action point

When you are next in placement, look out for advance care planning documentation. Is the Preferred Priorities for Care (PPC) tool used in your area?

Should patients wish to refuse specific medical treatments, for example cardio-pulmonary resuscitation or tube feeding, they can make an advance decision to refuse treatment. Further explanation of this is given in Chapter 4.

Supporting someone who doesn't feel able to cope with their dying relative at home

You may recall that Chapter 1 discussed the emphasis on the needs of the family as part of end-of-life care. This section will consider the assessment and care of close family members facing the prospect of a loved one who is being discharged from hospital and is expected to die at home.

Generally, relatives in this position may face a very difficult dilemma. They may perhaps feel caught between their desire to support and uphold their relatives' wishes in the remaining days of their life and anxieties concerning the emotional and practical consequences of caring at home (both for themselves and for their sick relative). Clearly the anxieties of carers can be multifaceted, and they may have a variety of concerns. As the end of life approaches, witnessing the decline of a loved one can be very distressing (Koop and Strang 2003). Some carers may find it hard to leave behind the reassurance and security of the hospital environment. And, of course, relatives may be anticipating the impending loss of their loved one and may have fears about the life they will have when they are bereaved. Others may be concerned about how the growing dependence of their loved one on them will limit their own enjoyment of life. Koop and Strang (2003) found this in their study of the experiences of carers of those dying from cancer, and Hasson et al. (2010) found this in their study of families caring for people with Parkinson's disease.

As we can see, Mrs Sevim is not unusual in being concerned about her husband being discharged home. It is important to assess her particular concerns as an individual. Discussing Mrs Sevim's concerns alongside her husband may increase their awareness of each other's anxieties and therefore their ability to offer mutual support. However, if it appears that Mrs Sevim is reluctant to disclose the worries she has about caring for her husband, it may be appropriate to offer her the opportunity to share her fears separately. This would enable her to speak freely about sensitive issues she does not wish to raise in her husband's presence. For example, she may have concerns about being at home with him after he has died and feel uncomfortable about mentioning this.

In Chapter 3 the importance of picking up cues, or hints, about patients' concerns was explored. In this case, Mrs Sevim has repeated her wish not to undertake personal care. This is an important cue so Helen should acknowledge this, give Mrs Sevim the opportunity to say more and then look for any other concerns to assess her needs. For example:

Helen: I understand that you are not able to wash and change your husband. Are there other things that it would be hard for you to do?

Later in the conversation Helen might ask: 'Is there anything else that is worrying you about your husband being at home?'

Reflective question

Clearly, relatives may have a whole range of anxieties when faced with the challenge of caring for a dying relative at home. Brainstorm as many possible fears as you can imagine that Mrs Sevim may have.

Mrs Sevim may hold a number of concerns. Below are just a few possibilities of anxious thoughts she may be having:

- How can I leave him to go to the shops?
- I find it so upsetting to see him so weak that I have to try hard not to cry when I visit him in hospital. Will I manage when we are at home together all the time?
- My friend Farah wanted to die at home but she was in agony so her daughter-in-law called for an ambulance. She died outside Casualty in great pain and surrounded by strangers. I don't want this to happen to Ahmed.

- He will not manage the stairs for the loo and I am not strong enough to help him.
- What do I do if something happens in the night?
- How am I going to manage the shop when he dies?

Once Helen has a full understanding of Mrs Sevim's worries and fears she is in a strong position to support Mrs Sevim successfully.

Reflective questions

Having considered the situation from Mrs Sevim's point of view, how might Helen support Mrs Sevim?

You may like to consider each of the following approaches, though you may also have ideas of your own.

- Helen could plan care services so that Mrs Sevim's care burden is as light as possible.
- Helen could refer Mrs Sevim to services that can offer her support.
- Helen could try to persuade Mr Sevim to accept care in some kind of institution (hospital, hospice or care home) as the care burden would otherwise be too much for Mrs Sevim.

Supporting someone daunted by the prospect of caring for a sick relative at home requires using the communication skills described in Chapter 3. It is imperative that nurses and health carers acknowledge the specific difficulties the relative faces and convey caring empathy in a genuine manner. Examples of phrases that might achieve this include:

- I can see the situation is difficult. What is it in particular that is worrying you about your husband coming home?
- You seem really worried he might fall at home. Is that right?

Once the concerns have been established, practical steps should be taken and advice should be offered to address issues that can be resolved or ameliorated. At the same time it should be acknowledged that some aspects of the situation cannot be changed and will remain difficult. The support in place to mitigate these difficulties needs to be clear, as do the limitations of what can be achieved. Examples of phrases which might achieve this include:

- We can provide extra pain relief in the home that he can take if his regular dose is insufficient.
- We can give the ambulance service information about your husband's condition so they will know about his illness and wishes should he fall at home and you need to call them in the night.
- District nurses and Macmillan nurses will visit you at home to support you alongside your husband.

Attempting to persuade Mr Sevim to accept institutional care is not respecting his wishes in respect of the principles set out in the Mental Capacity Act 2005 (Department of Constitutional Affairs 2007). Encouraging the couple to share their concerns may help them share their anxieties and make decisions that incorporate both their perspectives. Certainly, minimising the care that Mrs Sevim needs to provide is likely to be helpful, as is referring her to appropriate support services who can offer emotional support.

Clearly end-of-life care of patients at home is much more likely to be successful if carers' needs are addressed (Bee et al. 2008). Without proper assessment, incorrect assumptions can be made about the practical care they can offer and about the expectations that they have. If the assessment and preparation of carers has been comprehensive, carers should be better equipped to cope and be supported in their role.

Planning the care of someone whose needs are changing

Helen's apprehension concerning planning the discharge to home of Mr Sevim is understandable as he has complex needs. However, Helen has a good understanding of his present care needs and home situation, both of which are currently stable, so she is well placed to arrange his care at home. To plan his discharge well however, she also needs to anticipate the needs he may develop in future at home.

Generally, Helen should anticipate that Mr Sevim's fatigue, weakness and weight loss will worsen over the next few days or weeks leaving him increasingly debilitated. He is at risk of falling and may have very limited ability to look after himself. It is likely that he will become unable to bear weight in the near future and may need to be nursed in bed. Helen needs to consider how Mr Sevim's toileting needs can be met. While currently he may be able to use a commode by his bed, in the future he may need to be nursed in bed and require a urinal. Helen will need to refer to a service that can meet these practical care needs throughout a 24-hour period. She will also need to ensure that equipment such as a commode, urinal and possibly a hospital bed is available for Mr Sevim at home.

Changes in eating habits and weight loss can be a source of considerable distress within families, as eating and food preparation are often ways that families express their love and enjoy time together. Food can also be perceived as a source of much needed strength so that, if it is rejected, relatives can be deeply upset, causing tension (Hopkinson et al. 2006). Given that Mrs Sevim is most comfortable with shopping and food preparation, she may struggle as Mr Sevim eats less and less. Helen could consider ways to prepare Mrs Sevim for this, perhaps by gently explaining that diminishing appetite and eating is part of the illness and that sadly food will not make him feel stronger as she may hope.

While Mr Sevim's pain is currently controlled, it may extend in the future. If so, his analgesia (pain control medication) will need to be titrated (balanced) against his pain, as described in Chapter 6. Similarly, his breathlessness may worsen and require additional palliative treatment. This is described further in Chapter 6.

As Mr Sevim's disease advances he may develop some of the additional complications associated with advanced lung cancer. For example, since Mr Sevim's lung cancer has spread to his bones, he may develop pathological fractures, in that his diseased bones may break spontaneously or very easily. Should his cancer affect his spinal cord he may develop spinal cord compression, in which case diagnosis and treatment would be urgently required in order to prevent paralysis. Lung cancer can metastasise (spread) to the brain, causing a number of symptoms such as seizures (fits).

In addition to his practical care needs, there are therefore a number of potential problems that may compound Mr Sevim's current needs as he declines. He will need monitoring once he is at home and he may need specialist palliative care advice and treatment. Helen will need to refer him to a service that can offer such care.

The services available to people who need end-of-life care at home

A number of different services are available to care for dying patients and their relatives in their own homes. In this section they will be described so that we can consider which may be applicable to Mr and Mrs Sevim.

Most health care professionals offer end-of-life care to some of their patient group as part of their role using the palliative care approach (discussed in Chapter 5). These include ward-based nurses, social workers and occupational therapists, but district nurses and general practitioners (GPs) in particular have a central role in providing such care to those in their own homes.

There are a number of specialist palliative care providers in the community. These are practitioners who specialise exclusively in end-of-life care and hold specialist qualifications that reflect this. Many are based in hospices or specialist palliative care centres, but others may be based within hospitals or NHS Community Trusts. Hospice provision is widespread across the UK but varies hugely in terms of the provision offered. The roles of specialist palliative home care providers, and the integration of their roles with each other and generalist palliative care providers, is often complex and can be confusing for patients and families. Consequently, it is vital that health care professionals always become familiar with what it is available locally.

The charity Help the Hospices manages a directory of all hospices and palliative care services within the United Kingdom and Ireland as well as an international directory of hospice and palliative care services. Both directories are available free of charge online.

Action point

Have a look at the Directory of Hospice and Specialist Palliative Care Services at www.helpthehospices.org.uk/about-hospice-care/find-a-hospice/uk-hospice-and-palliative-care-services/. Which services are available in your local area?

The following information details the key types of community-based specialist palliative care providers available to patients at home.

Clinical nurse specialists in palliative/end-of-life care

Typically, clinical nurse specialists provide specialist advice and support on symptom control and psychosocial care to patients, families and generalist staff. They are likely to have education and research commitments to their role. They may work in the hospital or the community, or across the two settings. Clinical nurse specialists are managed in different ways. Some are attached to hospices; others are part of a Local Primary Care Trust or Acute Care Trust. Many are funded by or affiliated to the charity Macmillan Cancer Support and use the title Macmillan Nurse.

Hospice at home services

Many areas of the country have 'hospice at home' teams, although there is variation in how these are configured. Typically, these provide personal care and respite care in the home to enable families to have a break during the day or sleep at night. They may also support patients at home for short periods to prevent hospital discharge or enable early hospital discharge. These teams may be staffed by experienced care workers with some registered nurses.

Hospices

Hospice provision is widespread across the United Kingdom but varies hugely in terms of the provision offered. Hospices offer a range of specialist palliative care services including inpatient, day and community-based care. Patients are usually accepted for specialist care because of complex needs that cannot be met by generalist services, such as challenging symptoms or family circumstances. For example, they may have young children who are perhaps unaware of their diagnosis.

Multidisciplinary teams

A number of multidisciplinary specialist palliative/end-of-life care professionals are likely to be available to patients at home as and when they are required. Consultants in palliative medicine working with specialist registrars in palliative medicine offer medical assessment and management of patient with complex needs. Physiotherapy, occupational therapy, chaplaincy and social work are also commonly available. These services may be offered from a hospital, hospice or community service.

Inpatient specialist palliative care

Many hospices have inpatient beds available. These are likely to be for short stays of around two weeks for terminal care or symptoms assessment and control from a specialist multidisciplinary team. Access to hospice beds is usually determined by the needs of the patients; those with complex needs that are difficult to manage in other settings taking priority. Some hospices are able to offer admission in an emergency, 24 hours a day. Specialist palliative inpatient care beds are also available in some hospitals.

Day-care specialist palliative care

Many hospices offer day-care services to patients. These provide health care and social activities in a group setting, aiming to improve patients' quality of life and provide respite for families and carers. Specialist palliative day care is also offered in a small number of hospitals.

Outpatient specialist palliative care

Some palliative care outpatient services exist in which patients can see a specialist palliative care consultant in a clinic setting. These may be hospital- or hospice-based. They can be particularly helpful to patients who are generally cared for by practitioners using a palliative care approach but who encounter a complex problem. An example might be challenging pain which requires specialist advice through consultation.

Bereavement services

Many hospices and specialist palliative care teams offer dedicated bereavement services for those who are particularly at risk following bereavement. They usually offer a short series of one-to-one counselling sessions. These may include services for children affected by the death of a parent or other primary carer. Some hospices run bereavement support groups in which relatives can meet each other to offer mutual social support.

Nursing care homes

Some nursing homes have beds specifically registered for palliative care. Nursing care homes may be supported by specialist clinical nurses and consultants or registrars in palliative medicine.

Action point

Next time you are in practice ask colleagues which services they are aware of that are available locally for patients like Mr Sevim who wish to be cared for and die at home.

Co-ordinating discharge planning

Given the complexity of services outlined above, discharge planning can need careful co-ordination. The co-ordination of complex discharges is configured differently according to the services available in each hospital, but may include rapid discharge integrated care pathways, NHS Continuing Care teams and discharge planning co-ordinators.

Integrated care pathways

Given the importance of discharging dying patients home quickly, many hospitals have developed rapid discharge integrated care pathways, often adapted from the Liverpool Care Pathway for the Dying Patient (see Further reading for the website address). Part of their role is to expedite rapid discharge (perhaps within a few hours) for those on an end-of-life care pathway. To access this service, patients would need to meet local end-of-life care pathway criteria that assess whether the patient is approaching death with a prognosis of days rather than the weeks. Mr Sevim would not meet this criterion.

Action point

Make enquiries at the hospital in which you are next placed. Is there a rapid discharge integrated care pathway for dying patients? If so, is it being used and how quickly can patients on it be discharged home?

NHS Continuing Care

NHS Continuing Care is ongoing health care funded by the NHS for those living in the community, either at home or in a care facility such as a nursing home. Some hospitals have continuing health care access teams *in situ* who can assess patients for such provision. Continuing Care can be fast-tracked for those who have a rapidly deteriorating, possibly terminal, condition so that their care needs within the community can be met quickly through a package of care. Once a recommendation for fast-track care has been made by a registered health care professional responsible for assessing, managing and providing care for that patient, Primary Care Trusts or the equivalent are responsible for responding without delay (Department of Health 2009). It is likely that Mr Sevim would meet the criterion for fast-track continuing care.

Discharge planning co-ordinators

In recognition of the importance of good discharge planning, many hospitals have discharge planning co-ordinators to oversee complex discharges to home. It may be appropriate to refer Mr Sevim to this service.

> ## Action point
>
> Referring to the case of Mr Sevim and having considered Mr and Mrs Sevim's needs, put yourself in Helen's shoes. Considering the end-of-life care services that are available, what referrals would you make to expedite a rapid discharge home for Mr Sevim? How would you go about ensuring those referrals are made? You may like to make notes on this and review it after reading the discussion on discharge planning below.

Mr Sevim may well benefit from referral to an occupational therapist who may undertake a home visit to assess his care needs there, often in conjunction with a physiotherapist. He will be eligible for NHS Continuing Care to provide funding and to co-ordinate a care package, and this should be applied on a fast-track basis. If a 'hospice at home' service is available locally, then he could be referred to it. It may be that they are able to offer rapid care that will enable him to be discharged urgently.

Primarily, Mr Sevim will be under the care of his local GP. District nurses will be providing his nursing care. They are likely to be able to supply equipment such as a commode, hoist, hospital bed, pressure-relieving mattress and syringe drivers.

Given his high dependency, they may be supported by palliative carers such as 'hospice at home', who will undertake practical personal care such as attention to personal hygiene, mouth-care, bowel and bladder care. They may be able to provide carers to avoid any need for Mrs Sevim to provide care during the night.

In view of his deteriorating condition and the likelihood that his symptoms will exacerbate in future, he may benefit from specialist palliative care services and should therefore be referred to specialist palliative care providers in the community. They will be able to provide proactive advice on his pain and symptom management, anticipating and planning ahead for problems. They should also be available to support Mr and Mrs Sevim emotionally. They can access medical specialists in palliative care and may be able to access hospice-based bereavement services to support Mrs Sevim.

If he is well enough to travel, Mr Sevim may benefit from palliative day care, which is available at many hospices. There his symptoms would be monitored and reviewed regularly, and Mrs Sevim would have respite from caring.

In order to arrange services at home, referrals to all the above services will be required. Referral processes will vary in different areas but it is vital that complete and detailed information is given to enable community practitioners to be effective. Community services will need to know of Mr Sevim's preferred priorities for care and any 'advance decision' to refuse treatment he may have made.

Once referrals have been made, the ward nursing team needs to remain actively in touch to ascertain when services can commence. Ambulance transport will be required. The ambulance service will need to know of his Preferred Priorities for Care document, any advance decision to refuse treatment he may have made and any 'do not attempt cardiopulmonary resuscitation' order that has been agreed. Mr Sevim will also need a supply of his medication to take home.

Co-ordinating end-of-life care in the community

Given the plethora of services involved, it is not surprising that the co-ordination of end-of-life care in the community can be problematic. In particular, care offered outside normal working hours is limited in availability (Department of Health 2008) and co-ordination of care across different organisations, such as community nursing teams and ambulance clinicians, can be difficult.

In 2000, Dr Keri Thomas, a general practitioner, developed a system to co-ordinate and improve the quality of end-of-life care in the community. This is known as the Gold Standards Framework (GSF) (Thomas 2003) and has been implemented in many parts of the United Kingdom. It has been endorsed within the End of Life Care Strategy (Department of Health 2008) and has been strongly evaluated (Shaw et al. 2010). The Gold Standards Framework identifies patients who are likely to die in the next year by using trajectories or pathways that are generally experienced by a group of patients. This is done in conjunction with practitioners considering whether they would be surprised if the patient died within the next year. This is commonly known as the 'surprise question' and is described in Chapter 5. Once identified, patients are added to a register of end-of-life care patients. Often this is colour-coded in a traffic light system indicating the level of need of the patient, red being for patients like Mr Sevim who are very sick. Patients on the register are then discussed at monthly multidisciplinary meetings attended by GPs, district nurses, clinical nurse specialists in palliative care, and possibly others such as occupational therapists and paramedics. The meeting ensures that everyone is informed, allows discussion of difficult issues among the team, and offers a chance to reflect and learn from previous practice. A number of clinical tools in end-of-life care are available through the Gold Standards Framework website to support primary care teams to deliver quality end-of-life care (see Further reading for the website address). A key worker may be appointed from among the team members to co-ordinate the patient's care. Patients who are not receiving proactive services can also be monitored.

While not every primary health care team uses the Gold Standards Framework system, its principles of good teamworking and co-ordination are not unique and can be applied throughout. When considering discharging patients such as Mr Sevim, staff should identify whether the Gold Standards Framework has been adopted in the relevant primary health care team and, if so, they should request the patient be registered with it.

Action point

When you are next in community practice, find out whether the Gold Standards Framework is used in your area. You may wish to attend a multidisciplinary meeting.

Returning to Mr Sevim's Case

Helen and her ward nursing colleagues worked hard to ensure that Mr Sevim was able to be discharged home. Given his prognosis of a few weeks, he was not eligible for the hospital end-of-life care pathway. However, he was eligible for NHS Continuing Care. With the help of the continuing health care assessment team a comprehensive care package was arranged for Mr Sevim's arrival home, including a hospital bed and commode. He was referred both to local district nurses and clinical nurse specialists for ongoing symptom monitoring. With sensitive assessment, Mrs Sevim felt supported and, though she remained daunted, she was increasingly confident that she could manage.

Before he left the ward Mr Sevim made an advance care plan to refuse cardio-pulmonary resuscitation.

Fortunately, the primary care team where Mr Sevim lived used the Gold Standards Framework and Mr Sevim was placed on its supportive and palliative care register with his district nurse acting as key worker.

He remained at home until he died six weeks later.

Summary

The key points to remember when planning the discharge of someone to home when approaching the end of life include:

- Recognising and respecting the significance that being at home can have. Remember that very sick people, and indeed those living alone, can be cared for at home.
- Being realistic and honest about what care can be offered.
- The importance of assessing and supporting relatives and carers.
- Being cognisant of the range of community end-of-life care services available and how referral to them can be made and co-ordinated.

Further reading

Charlton, R. (ed.) (2002) *Primary Palliative Care: Dying, Death and Bereavement in the Community*. Abingdon: Radcliffe Medical Press.
This book is written particularly for those working in the community, and equips the reader with useful knowledge of end-of-life care in this setting. It includes chapters on out of hours and emergency care, and on the needs of informal carers. As such, it will give those working in the hospital setting an understanding of the context into which they are discharging patients.

Tadman, M. and Roberts, D. (2007) *Oxford Handbook of Cancer Nursing*. Oxford: Oxford University Press.
This is one of a number of books that describe the assessment of management of common cancers in an accessible way.

Lees, L. (2007) *Nurse-Facilitated Discharge*. Keswick: M & K Publishing.
Although not specific to end-of-life care, this book covers all aspects of discharging patients from hospital.

www.goldstandardsframework.org.uk/
This is the website for the Gold Standards Framework as discussed in the chapter.

www.helpthehospices.org.uk/hospiceinformation/
This is the website of Help the Hospices, which hosts the Directory of Hospice and Palliative Care Services discussed within the chapter.

www.mcpcil.org.uk/liverpool-care-pathway/
This is the website of the Liverpool Care Pathway for the Dying Patient.
www.endoflifecareforadults.nhs.uk/publications/ppcform

The Preferred Priorities for Care document is available on the End of Life Care Programme website at the link above.

References

Bee, P., Barnes, P. and Luker, K. (2008) 'A systematic review of informal caregivers' needs in providing home-based end-of-life care to people with cancer', *Journal of Clinical Nursing*, 18: 1379–93.

Department of Constitutional Affairs (2007) *The Mental Capacity Act 2005: Code of Practice*. London: The Stationery Office. Available online at: www.direct.gov.uk/prod_consum_dg/groups/dg_digitalassets/@dg/@en/@disabled/documents/digitalasset/dg_186484.pdf [accessed 22 April 2012].

Department of Health (2008) *End of Life Care: Promoting High Quality Care for All Adults at the End of Life*. London: DH.

Department of Health (2009) *The National Framework for NHS Continuing Healthcare and NHS-funded Nursing Care (revised)*. London: DH. Available online at: www.dh.gov.uk/prod_consum_dh/groups/dh_digitalassets/documents/digitalasset/dh_103161.pdf [accessed 3 August 2012].

Hasson, F., Kernohan, W.G., McLaughlin, M., Waldron, M., McLaughlin, D., Chambers, H. and Cochrane, B. (2010) 'An exploration into the palliative and end-of-life care experiences of carers of people with Parkinson's disease', *Palliative Medicine*, 24(7): 731–6.

Higginson, I. (2003) *Priorities and Preferences for End-of-Life Care in England, Wales and Scotland*. London: National Council for Hospice and Specialist Palliative Care Services.

Higginson, I.J. and Sen-Gupta, G.J.A. (2000) 'Place of care in advanced cancer: a qualitative systematic literature review of patient preferences', *Palliative Medicine*, 3(3): 287–300.

Hopkinson, J., Wright, D. and Corner, J. (2006) 'Exploring the experience on weight loss in people with advanced cancer', *Journal of Advanced Nursing*, 54(3): 304–12.

Koop, P. and Strang, V. (2003) 'The bereavement experience following home-based family care giving for persons with advanced cancer', *Clinical Nursing Research*, 12: 127–44.

Lees, L. (2007) *Nurse Facilitated Discharge from Hospital*. Keswick: M & K Publishing.

Munday, D., Dale, J. and Murray, S. (2007) 'Choice of death: individual preferences, uncertainty and the availability of care', *Journal of the Royal Society of Medicine*, 100: 211–15.

Shaw, K.L., Clifford, C., Thomas, K. and Meehan, H. (2010) 'Improving end-of-life care: a critical review of the Gold Standards Framework in primary care', *Palliative Medicine*, 24(3): 317–29.

Thomas, K. (2003) *Caring for the Dying at Home: Companions on the Journey*. Oxford: Radcliffe Medical Press Ltd.

Townsend, J., Frank, A.O., Fermont, D., Dyer, S., Karran, O., Walgrove, A. and Piper, M. (1990) 'Terminal cancer care and patients' preference for place of death: a prospective study', *British Medical Journal*, 301(6749): 415–17.

UK Parliament (2005) *The Mental Capacity Act 2005* [Act of Parliament]. London: The Stationery Office. Available online at: www.legislation.gov.uk/ukpga/2005/9/pdfs/ukpga_20050009_en.pdf [accessed 30 April 2012].

CHAPTER 8

Knowing when a patient is in the last days of life

Joanna De Souza

This chapter will explore:

- What we mean by a 'good death'
- The common signs that someone is entering the last days of life
- End-of-life care pathways
- Managing patients in the last 48 hours of life
- The challenges of placing people on to an end-of-life care pathway
- Supporting the families and children of someone who is dying

Introduction

Working in health care, we will often be working with patients who are extremely unwell for a variety of reasons. Usually these people will recover if given the appropriate treatment and our role as nurses is to monitor and assist these patients to recovery. However, some of the patients we care for will not recover and learning to recognise when a patient is dying is a life-long journey and sometimes even the most experienced practitioners get it wrong. Nevertheless, there are patterns of behaviour and physiological signs that, with experience, we learn to recognise and that allow us to make reasonable judgements about when people are at the end of life. This chapter will explore those clues and discuss how we may approach care delivery at this time. Through better recognition of the signs of dying, it is hoped that many more patients may be able to benefit from the tools and interventions that now exist to make the process of dying a more comfortable one.

The following case study offers an example of when an inpatient hospital team may want to involve a specialist palliative care team into a patient's plan of care. This chapter will use this situation to explore some of the decision-making that goes on in these situations.

Reg

Mr Peters, Reg, as he is known, has had congestive cardiac failure for several years, and has been managing with support in his sheltered accommodation. However, over the past few months, Reg has been admitted into hospital three times following episodes of severe chest pain and increasing swelling of his feet (oedema). Investigations have shown that his kidney function is also deteriorating. His last discharge was only three weeks ago. When he came into hospital this time he was very weak and confused. Even after intravenous medications had been started, he remained drowsy and mildly confused. You have been looking after him for two days now and you notice that he is slowly becoming less easy to rouse and he is really struggling to eat or drink. Often when someone has been helping him with some soft diet, he only swallows it with difficulty and, if not encouraged, food will remain un-swallowed in his mouth. When drinking he often chokes slightly and it makes him splutter and cough. You have referred him to the speech therapist to check his swallowing reflex. He is getting weaker and is unable to cough properly. His mouth is becoming harder to clean and his tongue appears to be coated with a white film. During the ward round your mentor suggests that it may be appropriate to put Reg onto the integrated care pathway for the dying as he now fulfils two of the criteria, i.e. he is bed bound and only taking sips of fluid. The cardiac team agree. However, Reg is not really able to have a discussion so the team decide to discuss it with his family when they come in.

CASE STUDY

What we mean by a 'good death'

Before we go too far into the details of how to offer good symptom control and make our patients comfortable, it is important to consider what it is that makes for a 'good death'. Reflection on this will help us to prioritise the care that we offer to our patients and their families. Jones (2007) reminds us that a good death is one that is appropriate for and requested by that particular patient. Drawing on the report by Henwood and Neuberger (1999) for Age Concern on 'The Future of Health and Care of Older People', Burns (2010) highlighted that the themes of control, autonomy and independence emerge constantly in the debate of what makes for a good death. Their report outlines 12 guiding principles to constitute a good death which include elements such as the importance of knowing when death is coming and having some understanding of what may be expected even in situations when prognostication is more complicated. They included the importance of having time to say goodbye and perhaps some control over other aspects of timing. Their final guiding principle called for the enabling of people to be able to leave when it is time to go and not have life prolonged pointlessly.

Earlier chapters in this book have already considered how we can address some of these aspects earlier in the patient's illness journey.

For Reg at this stage, the major principles from this report which may be useful to consider when planning his care provision are: being afforded privacy and dignity, control of pain and other symptoms, to have control over who is present and can share the end, access to spiritual and psychological support and care and any specialist care he may require, and lastly to be able to leave when it is time to go and not have life prolonged.

The common signs that someone is entering the last days of life

As the body becomes overwhelmed with the burden of disease or multiple organs are no longer able to perform their normal functions, there are some general signs that indicate a patient is coming to the end of their lives. With many patients this will be a gradual process and is related to the gradual deterioration of the body systems. With some illnesses, treatable acute exacerbations of their disease may present similar symptoms so accurate assessment is required. The National Cancer Institute (2010) offers a useful breakdown, with some helpful information that allows relatives and friends to understand what the signs are. For example:

- Drowsiness.
- Confusion as the body's electrolytes become imbalanced.
- Reduced urine output as kidney function declines. The urine will often become dark as it becomes more concentrated.
- Increased breathlessness and loss of colour (cyanosis) as gas exchange in the lungs become less effective.
- Retained secretion in upper airways resulting in gurgling or rattling sounds.
- Breathlessness caused by reduction in blood flow thorough the cardiac system.
- Increasing amounts of peripheral oedema with the reduction of the production of plasma proteins such as albumin, which traditionally encourage the fluid to stay within the bloodstream rather than settling in the interstitial spaces in the body tissues.

When we start to see these signs and symptoms developing while caring for the patient, it is helpful to discuss them with family members so that they too can become prepared gradually, rather than when death is very imminent.

Reflective question

When caring for someone like Reg, who is dying, what do you feel would make a good death for him?

What factors do you think may most influence Reg's death?

End-of-life care pathways

Managing the last days of life has been a major focus of palliative care guidance in the past few years, including a national rolling out of an integrated care pathway for the end of life, initially known as the Liverpool Care Pathway (LCP). This tool, developed by two experienced palliative care practitioners, suggests a series of criteria to help practitioners to recognise when death is very near and possibly within the next 48 hours (Ellershaw and Wilkinson 2003). The LCP has been adapted in some Trusts to reflect local policies and it is often known as end-of-life care pathways (ECPs). The pathways are designed to be used with patients who are:

- bed bound;
- semi-comatose;
- only able to take sips of fluid;
- no longer able to take tablets.

Our patient, Reg, is displaying the signs characteristic of the end of life. He remains drowsy, is becoming less easy to rouse and often chokes slightly when drinking. Despite him having had intravenous medications to try to treat reversible causes such as infection, he has continued to deteriorate, so it would seem appropriate to consider starting him on the pathway.

The components of the pathway are covered in the following three steps:

1. Initial assessment

The pathway divides this assessment into four areas.

- Comfort measures such as pain, nausea, etc.
- Psychological insights, such as seeking to ascertain the patient's understanding of their condition and what is happening to them.
- Spiritual support, including assessment of religious needs and important rituals.
- Communication, which includes determining the understanding of the family and notifying other members of the health care team of the patient's current condition (e.g. his or her GP).

2. Ongoing care

Using the assessment, a plan of care can be made. The pathway recommends frequent reassessment, particularly of symptom control measures. It is recommended
that reassessment is carried out every four hours in the acute setting and at reasonable, but again frequent, regularity in primary care settings.

3. Care of the family and carers after death

An ECP lays out a series of goals to offer well-organised but sensitive care to people
at this very difficult time. Traditionally, care after death has been delivered in an
ad hoc way due to fluctuating levels of specialist provision and lack of confidence
on the part of nurses.

Placing someone on an ECP takes very careful decision-making and collaborative
practice. Initially, it is important to do a thorough assessment to determine whether
the ECP approach is suitable in the situation and for the patient. To go back to our
case study, sadly it would be difficult to include Reg in the decision-making process.
However, if he had made an advanced care plan, this would need to be taken into
consideration and it is imperative to involve his relatives and next of kin.

Most clinical areas, either acute hospitals or community settings, have developed
an end-of-life care pathway for use in this area. Most will be based on and remain
similar to the Liverpool Care Pathway.

Table 8.1 illustrates the start of the initial assessment. This continues to cover
issues such as who has been informed and other communication issues. The pathway
documentation then enables a more complete symptom assessment to be made and
documented. It concludes with a pathway for the declaration, verification and communication of the death itself and matters relating to the care of bereaved relatives.

The pathway documentation offers suggestions for care decisions and recommends
that should different care decisions be made (they call these variances), these will be

Table 8.1   A sample pathway document (Ellershaw and Wilkinson, 2003)

	Patient assessment	
Diagnosis	Date of admission	Ethnicity
Physical condition		
Comfort measures	Goal 1: Current medication assessed and non-essentials discontinued	
	Goal 2: PRN subcutaneous medication written up for list below as per protocol	
	Goal 3: Discontinue inappropriate interventions	
	Decisions to discontinue inappropriate nursing interventions taken	

documented, with the rationale for the decisions, so that all members of the team are clear about the direction being taken. Ellershaw and Wilkinson (2003) discuss some of the elements that may be changing, such as the need for a discussion about cardio-pulmonary resuscitation and the discontinuation of unnecessary interventions such as artificial hydration. We will look at this in more detail later in this chapter.

Action point

Identify the ECP used in your area of practice. Read and become familiar with it and identify any elements that raise questions for you. Discuss these with the clinical area palliative care link person or a member of the local specialist palliative care team.

Managing patients in the last 48 hours of life

When someone is within the last 48 hours of their life, the ECP prompts the monitoring of the following common symptoms: pain, agitation, respiratory tract secretions, nausea and vomiting, stomatitis and urinary difficulties. It then provides space to add additional symptoms that may be specific to that patient. Let us look at the management of Reg's symptoms.

On initial assessment Reg is having increasingly severe chest pain and oedema, difficulty with swallowing and dysphasia. As his pulmonary oedema increases, he will also have problems with dysnoea. He remains confused and drowsy.

Pain management

At this stage, as is common at this stage of life, it is becoming increasingly difficult for Reg to take his medications, such as his cardiac medications, his diuretics and his analgesia. The emphasis of care at this stage is to increase comfort as much as possible. As pharmacological management is a major tool in this area, it may be appropriate to consider the use of a syringe driver using low doses of morphine for pain control and dyspnoea, together with a benzodiazipine such as midazolam. It may also be helpful to consider continuing a loop diuretic such as frusamide (Littlewood and Johnson 2006) also via the subcutaneous route.

In 2008 the Department of Health published guidelines for prescribing in advanced chronic kidney disease. These guidelines were devised by the team developing the Liverpool Care Pathway and a renal steering group, and are very useful in guiding what should be in the syringe driver.

Prescribing for people with end-stage cardiac disease is complex and not all medications can be given by syringe driver. Good collaboration may be required between the cardiac team, the specialist palliative care team and the pharmacists and careful thought needs to go into which medications are really making a difference to their symptom control at this stage. Medications that have a longer term aim, such as cholesterol lowering medications etc., can be discontinued. Often medications that patients have needed previously, such as drugs controlling high blood pressure or blood clotting, may not be necessary as due to the patient's lack of mobility and reduced fluid intake, their blood pressure may be low and their blood counts may be falling.

The *Changing Gear* guidelines produced by the National Council for Palliative Care (2006) suggest that when reviewing medications at this stage of a patient's life only medications aimed at preventing distressing symptoms should be continued. The following categories cover the main types of drug that will be needed at this time:

1   Analgesics – for pain.
2   Anxiolytics – to relieve distress.
3   Anti-secretories – to relieve upper respiratory tract secretions that can impede comfortable breathing.
4   Anti-emetics – to relieve nausea and vomiting.

Action point

Patients may have been on some of their medications for many years and relatives can find it very difficult when there is discussion of discontinuing these medications at this stage. It is important to be aware of this and it can be useful to ask the nurse looking after the patient to discuss the rationale with them.

Mouth care

As people become less well and are less able to take oral fluids, they become dehydrated and one of the side-effects of this is a very dry mouth which then becomes vulnerable to breakdown and subsequent infection. This is usually indicative of what is happening throughout the gastrointestinal (GI) tract. There are a number of reasons for this, including a breakdown in the body's ability to process and eliminate waste products as the major organs start to shut down. This results in an increase of waste material being carried around in the bloodstream so normal cell maintenance processes slow down, such as the production of saliva and its cleansing components, and blood cells that help to repair the GI tract from its normal wear and tear.

Reg's mouth is becoming harder to clean and his tongue appears to be coated with a white film. Regular assessment of the whole oral cavity is important and should be done every two to three hours. With Reg, because of his breathing difficulties and potential oxygen therapy, he will require assistance with his mouth more frequently and some type of hydrating intervention should be offered hourly.

The white appearance of Reg's tongue may well indicate a candidiasis infection. Candidiasis is a fungal infection more commonly known as thrush. It can be treated with antifungal agents such as Nystatin suspension or fluconazole if Reg is able to swallow this. Oral candidiasis is often a sign that candidiasis may be present further down the GI tract and may cause some swallowing discomfort and in some cases diarrhoea. It is important, where possible, to get Reg to swallow his liquid medication (suspension) and to refrain from rinsing his mouth for about half an hour after administration.

The use of an oral care protocol and monitoring sheet can be really helpful here in ensuring details are kept and regular care is given. A good example is the protocol formulated by the Accord hospice (Milligan et al. 2001).

Terminal restless

Sometimes referred to as terminal delirium, not only is this a difficult symptom both to observe and to manage with a patient and family, but it is also difficult in terms of the decision-making that needs to take place. It is an acute confusional state that is characterised by fluctuating periods of consciousness. Patients often present as behaving inappropriately, being unaware of place and time, being agitated, and being liable to harm themselves. It is a very common symptom occurring in between 85% and 90% of patients at the very end of life (Moyer 2011). A lack of understanding of this symptom often causes a level of distress, particularly in relatives. It can be very distressing and exhausting to observe and leaves carers in a position of being unable to meet the needs of the patient (Brajtman 2005).

Kyle (2009) discusses a number of reversible causes of terminal agitation that it is important to exclude, such as blocked catheters, thirst or poor pain control. Moyer (2011) offers a detailed approach to clear assessment and diagnosis of this condition and its management, which it may be useful to consider, particularly in elderly patients. However, this type of detailed assessment is not always possible when patients are at this stage in end-of-life care due to their overall deteriorating health. This is the case with Reg. Anxiolytics such as haloperidol, which does not cause deep sedation and has a wide therapeutic range, are commonly used. They can be titrated and given either orally or in injectable or suppository form (Kyle 2009).

In her exploration of delirium management, Kyle (2009) also discusses the concern that arises about the relationship between the control of these difficult symptoms, such as delirium and agitation, and the perception that symptom control at the end of life is being used to hasten death. She acknowledges that it remains a challenging situation to get the level of sedation right and to ensure that it is undertaken with good communication with families and other professionals involved.

Noisy breathing

This can be one of the most distressing symptoms for carers at the end of life. It can be colloquially known as a 'death rattle', partly as it often arises near to the death event. Although the patient may appear to be unaware of their breathing as they may be semi-conscious, for the carers it is an omnipresent sound that, like a young baby's cry, is difficult to listen to unresponsively. Noisy breathing can be due to a number of factors but most commonly it is generally accepted that the noisy respirations are heard when the dying person can no longer clear their airways.

Clark and Butler (2009) suggest that better understanding and assessment of the cause as well as determining the positioning of the fluid causing the problem can lead to better care. They offer a number of strategies for dealing with the symptom, starting with repositioning of the patient using the bed back and pillows. Turning patients can often redistribute fluid accumulation and allow for easier breathing for a period of time. Gentle suctioning can also be used to remove pooled fluid in the mouth and upper respiratory tract.

There are a number of pharmacological interventions in common practice for the management of noisy breathing, the most common being anticholinergic medications such as hyoscine hydrobromide. However, the systematic review conducted by Wee and Hillier (2008) demonstrates that this is a poorly researched area which depends far more on traditional practices than research evidence. Currently there is little evidence that these medications work better than placebos.

The challenges of placing people on to an end-of-life care pathway

Making the decision that someone has reached the very end stages of life and may be heading into their last weeks of life is known as 'diagnosing dying'. The practitioners that devised the Liverpool Care Pathway (Ellershaw and Wilkinson 2003) caution that predicting that someone is in the dying phases of a disease such as cancer is recognised to be an easier task than with patients dying of chronic diseases, such as chronic airways disease and end stage heart disease. This is because the processes move more slowly so the degree of deterioration is harder to detect and recognise. It is therefore important to ensure that a full assessment is made by an experienced medical practitioner before deciding to place a patient on an end-of-life care pathway.

In reality, many patients are not diagnosed as dying early enough. When Gibbins et al. (2009) carried out an audit looking at deaths that occurred in an acute hospital and when they were predicted, they found that 87% of patients dying in the setting were recognised as dying less than 72 hours prior to death. Their conclusion was that diagnosing dying was difficult for clinicians working in a setting where patients may come close to death and then pull through and where cure is the major focus and in some sense death is still viewed as some sort of failure. They also suggested that more research is needed to identify diagnostic signs of death, and that we need to work harder at creating an environment where cure is not seen as the ultimate aim in all situations. Instead, a palliative care approach can run alongside active management.

Symptom control or assisted dying?

Another challenge of using an end-of-life care pathway is the concern that it may be a prescription for euthanasia as it does support the use of adequate pain relief and sedation to control symptoms of agitation and delirium. A series of articles run in *The Daily Telegraph* in 2009 by two journalists included headings such as 'Sentenced to death on the NHS', 'Daughter claims father wrongly placed on controversial NHS end of life scheme' (Devlin 2009; Irvine and Devlin 2009). The articles discussed anxieties by both families and clinicians that the tool may be used too prescriptively and people may be denied potentially life-promoting interventions. Events such as these highlight the importance of the careful and open communication that there needs to be among professionals and with patients and families when we are considering putting someone on the LCP, including explanation and discussion of the plan as well as the careful use of these tools to *assist* practice rather than to dictate practice. Review of the patient's condition may indicate that some symptoms have resolved and it is important to remove them from the pathway if they are no longer thought to be in the last 48 hours of life.

How long can someone survive who is no longer eating and drinking?

Something that often causes a great deal of anxiety to both friends and relatives, and also to staff, is how the patient will feel when they can no longer swallow to eat and drink. This anxiety often results in patients being started on intravenous fluids and sometimes artificial feeding while these decisions are being considered.

Potentially the use of artificial hydration using intravenous fluids (IV hydration) at the end of life may help to relieve the patient's dry mouth. However, it can also result in increased difficulties with a build-up of secretions, an increased need for catheterisation and a build-up of oedema as the body's ability to regulate the fluid balance of the body deteriorates (Bavin 2007). The National Council for Palliative Care's *Artificial Nutrition and Hydration* guidance document (2007) discusses how subjecting a body that is having difficulty processing its bodily functions to artificial feeding may lead to an increase in discomfort such as tissue oedema, excess production of urine and faecal matter which can result in constipation or diarrhoea.

Assessing whether a patient is uncomfortable because of thirst or dehydration, or the increased load on failing major organs, or the distress of incontinence when in the last days of life is a difficult call to make. The most important factor is to not have blanket rules but to assess the needs of each patient and to ensure assessment is an ongoing process. IV hydration can be useful in symptom control, for example in the management of urinary tract infection.

All too often it becomes the policy of a practice area that decides the outcome. Often in acute units there is a tendency to hydrate and in specialist units such as hospices a tendency not to. A common issue that arises in acute inpatient settings is that patients are routinely initiated on to IV fluids as they are admitted, often in the accident and emergency department and perhaps before a full understanding of their level of deterioration has been established.

Careful consideration of a patient's prognosis before commencing IV hydration or feeding can alleviate much suffering in the long term for patient, family and professional care givers. Taking down an intravenous infusion because it is not in patient's best interest is a much harder decision and action for a family and team than not starting one in the first place. However, if it does not seem appropriate for that patient, reducing or discontinuing parental fluid at this stage can be easier for families if they can see the potential problem it is causing and why it is unlikely to be resolved.

Although they note that the evidence is conflictive, Clark and Butler (2009) suggest that limited use of parental hydration, such as is seen in specialist palliative care units, does seem to be effective. Individual assessments and effective discussion among the health care team and the patient's carers is really important in helping to make this decision.

The issue of hydration and feeding at the end of life has been a contentious one for many years and remains a very difficult issue over which there is still much debate. Such decisions are rarely easy for families or the health care professionals involved. Much of the palliative care literature offers compelling arguments against it and the National Council for Palliative Care (2007) has produced some clear guidelines that can be used to guide practice.

Supporting the families and children of someone who is dying

If we return to our patient Reg, his story illustrates the situations that often occur, and explores how we might handle them and the discussions that may arise.

CASE STUDY

Reg (2)

Reg's daughter, Olive (his next of kin), visits Reg in the early afternoon. You approach her and after some general conversation suggest that it would be useful for her to have a chat in the sister's office with you, the nurse looking after Reg, and the doctor about how Reg is getting on. She agrees, saying that it would be really helpful to be able to talk things through as she has been worried about him.

When the doctor is free, together you discuss Reg's continual deterioration with Olive. She has also noticed and was aware that Reg had been getting progressively unwell over the past few months. You explain that it appears that Reg may be reaching the end of life and discuss some of the signs you have been observing. Although she says that in many ways they have been expecting this, she is quite upset and becomes tearful. You are able to sit with her quietly and allow her to talk through how sad it feels. When Olive asks what is likely to happen now, your mentor discusses the integrated care pathway and its aim of allowing people to have a dignified death. You are all able to talk about what this may mean for Reg.

One of Olive's major concerns is that if Reg does not have an intravenous feeding he may starve to death.

If Reg had made any kind of advanced care plan (discussed in Chapter 4), we would need to abide by it to respect his autonomy of person. However, in the absence of an advanced care plan, we need to consider the balance between maleficence and non-maleficence, i.e. between the need to offer care in the best interest of the patient and the imperative that we must do no harm to the patient.

While answering any questions, and addressing concerns, this gives us an opportunity to prepare families for what to expect over the next few days. Below is an example of the potential conversation around this topic.

Olive: One other thing, what I am very worried about is that dad might starve to death. This morning he didn't have any breakfast. I tried to help him with some porridge but he wouldn't swallow any of it.

Nurse: Yes your dad is getting weaker and he is now really struggling to eat and drink.

Olive: It has been two days since he has eaten anything really. I think he needs to be fed by a drip.

Nurse: Olive, it is very distressing to see Reg becoming so weak. However, it is not the lack of food that is causing it. Reg's body is slowing down. In the advanced stage of his disease, because his heart is no longer able to pump his blood round effectively, his other organs, such as his kidneys and liver, are not getting the blood supply they need. Because of this, these organs cannot do their jobs either, so any food and drink that Reg is having may not be able to be processed anyway. This is a sign that people may be moving into the last few days of life.

Before we think of putting up a drip we have to think about whether it will make your dad feel better or worse. It may cause him more problems as it may make fluid build up in the wrong places and cause breathing difficulties.

What is really important at this stage is keeping Reg as comfortable as possible. Keeping his mouth and lips moist, keeping his skin moist so that it doesn't crack and leave him vulnerable to infection are really key things. I wonder if you would be able to take responsibility for those and, using the equipment we will give you, to regularly give him sips of water and mouth washes and cream his limbs. You will need to be very gentle with his legs as you can see they are quite swollen with the fluid that is gathering.

Olive [weeping gently]: Oh yes, I see. You are right, I can see he is getting more poorly. It is just so hard to accept he won't get better and that we really are getting near the end.

However, I have some lovely cream at home. I will bring that in for his feet, I did notice the heels were starting to look cracked, that might make them feel more comfortable.

[Small silence]

Nurse: That will be great, Olive. It is good to talk about anything that any of you are concerned about.

This becomes a more difficult conversation to have when it seems appropriate to stop IV hydration that is already ongoing. However, it is important that the conversation does take place and is not left until someone more senior is available to discuss it. Time is so limited in these situations. Again, careful explanations with the family and suggestions that they become involved with looking after and assessing Reg's comfort may enable them to work through their anxieties by playing a more active role.

As can be seen from the example above, discussing the signs of imminent death with friends and relatives before and as they occur is vitally important. Family members are often concerned about the changes they observe, but they seldom know the right questions to ask to make sense of the process of death. Developing a relationship with them and having frequent conversations allows families to express their fears and worries and also allows you to start to prepare them so that the death of their relatives is not such a sudden and unexpected event for them.

These conversations also allow the opportunity to start to explore issues around place of death. If started early enough, this enables families to make more informed choices, for example, about taking their relative home to die.

What about children?

Involving children in the process of dying is one that causes very mixed views. When it is the child who is dying, this is a specialised area of care, and there are useful books and resources for developing an understanding of the needs in that area which are outside the remit of this book. Rolls (2008) offers a very useful chapter on the needs of children and it would be worth reading this to help you understand more on this topic.

However, when it is children who have links with the person who is dying, their experiences are very often shaped by where the dying process is taking place. When someone dies at home, or in a specialist centre such as a hospice, children are often involved. This may be either through necessity because they are physically present, or through facilitation by specialists within the hospice or community setting. However, when the death is in hospital, it is often much more by chance that children are involved with the dying process.

It is common that people feel that children may be upset by watching someone they know die and that it is kinder to keep them out of the situation and allow them to get on with their own lives. At times it may appear that children do not get very affected by the serious illness of a family member. John Bowlby's work on attachment demonstrates a child's capacity to react to a separation involving a significant relationship from an early age (Bowlby 2005). Worden (2001) looks further at this concept of when children develop the capacity to mourn and finds that from as young as 3–4 years of age, children display mourning behaviours. Involving children in the dying process, like adults, allows them to start to explore the losses they are experiencing and the effect that the death will have on them. Chapter 11 looks in more detail at the way children handle loss. However, we need to think about how we involve children at the time of death to help them deal more effectively with their bereavement.

Reg's family

Olive, Reg's daughter, has three children – Alicia, a helpful 16 year-old, Linda, aged 5, and Michael, aged 7. They live in the same block of flats and were often looked after by their grandparents during holiday times and at weekends when their mum was busy, so they are very close to their grandfather. Since the death of their grandmother three years ago, their grandfather has become increasingly less able, although the children continued to visit regularly.

Since their grandfather has been in hospital, none of the children has been to visit. Olive felt it would be too stressful to bring the children and that they may be upset to see their grandfather looking so unwell. Alicia has had to increase her caring role for her siblings while her mother has been tied up at the hospital. Linda and Michael appear unaffected by their grandfather's deteriorating health. It is the school holidays and the children have not been able to get out very much as Olive is so busy visiting Reg. This has been difficult for everyone.

CASE STUDY

How can we care for these children?

The National Council for Palliative Care's *Dying Matters* (2012) campaign for more openness around dying urges an open approach to be taken with children to avoid misunderstandings and to offer the opportunity to acknowledge the losses being faced by children.

When Olive comes to visit Reg, it may be helpful to talk to her about the children. This may start as an initial enquiry about how they are getting on and sharing with her how complex it must be to manage them as well as visiting Reg in hospital. However, this conversation also gives us an opportunity to explore with her what she may have told the children and something about the importance of talking to children about death. If you are able to keep some appropriate leaflets in the wards, such as the *Dying Matters* leaflets, these can provide useful information for her to take away and consider.

Together with other members of the nursing team, it may be appropriate to offer support to Olive about having these conversations by suggesting that she bring the children in with her and one of the nurses can facilitate a conversation with them and Olive. If she does not feel happy to do this, she may prefer your help in preparing what she might say to the children herself when at home. It is much better to broach the subject even if one isn't sure what to say, rather than leave it because it is too difficult.

The candle project at St Christopher's Hospice (Kraus 2007) was set up to help both young people affected by death and those who work with the dying where there may be young people involved. Their helpful leaflet suggests that it is important to offer children:

- information about what has happened and why, and what is likely to happen next;
- reassurance that they are not to blame for what has happened and that they will be cared for;
- an opportunity to express their feelings and to make choices about their involvement in rituals such as the funeral;
- an opportunity to offer comfort as well as to receive it by encouraging adults to share their feelings with their children;
- help in dealing with bereavement as this can prevent serious problems later in life.

Marie Curie also produces some very helpful leaflets for staff and families, including leaflets specifically designed for different age groups of children. These are available through their website (Marie Curie 2012).

Summary

The key points to remember when caring for someone in the last days of life are:

- There are common signs that help us to recognise when someone is entering the last stages of life. Following discussion with the health care team, we should initiate appropriate measures to enable a good death.
- The end-of-life care pathways help us to work through the measures we need to consider at this point in a patient's disease trajectory.
- Symptom control in the last 48 hours of life often involves decisions about discontinuing medications and other interventions that are no longer contributing to the patient's comfort.
- Supporting the families of the person who is dying is a major part of our role at this stage. We may need to have discussions about difficult issues such as artificial nutrition and hydration at the end of life.
- All members of a family and social network will be affected by a death in the family. It is important to consider the needs of people who may sometimes be disenfranchised, such as children or ex-partners.

Further reading

Try to access your local copy of the end-of-life care pathway. Explore some of the areas it covers by referring to John Ellershaw and Suzie Wilkinson's book on the development and implementation of the Liverpool Care Pathway: Ellershaw, J. and Wilkinson, S. (2003) *Care of the Dying: A Pathway to Excellence*. Oxford: Oxford University Press.

It may be useful to look at the guidelines produced by the National Council for Palliative Care on the issue of artificial hydration and nutrition at the end of life and consider how this reflects your own feelings about this issue: National Council for Palliative Care (2007) *Artificial Nutrition and Hydration: Guidance in End of Life Care for Adults*. London: NCPC.

The film *Step Mom* (1998), directed by Chris Columbus and starring Julia Roberts and Susan Sarandon, offers an insightful picture of the needs of children when there is serious illness in the family and has a touching scene when the parents find they need to talk about the mother's illness with the children.

References

Bavin, L. (2007) 'Artificial rehydration in palliative care: is it beneficial?', *International Journal of Palliative Nursing*, 13(9): 445–9.

Bowlby, J. (2005) *A Secure Base* (re-issue). Oxford: Routledge.

Brajtman, S. (2005) 'Terminal restlessness: perspectives of an interdisciplinary palliative care team', *International Journal of Palliative Nursing*, 11(4): 170–8.

Burns, E. (2010) *Principles of a Good Death as Identified by Age Concern in Palliative and End-of-Life Care for Older People British Geriatrics Society* [online]. Available at: www.bgs.org.uk/index.php?option=com_content&view=article&id=368:palliativecare&catid =12:goodpractice&Itemid=106 [accessed 25 May 2012].

Clark, K. and Butler, M. (2009) 'Noisy respiratory secretions at the end of life', *Current Opinion in Supportive and Palliative Care*, 3(2): 120–4.

Department of Health (2008) *Liverpool Care Pathway (LCP) Guidelines for LCP Drug Prescribing in Advanced Chronic Kidney Disease*. London: DH.

Devlin, K. (2009) 'Sentenced to death on the NHS', *The Daily Telegraph*, 2 September.

Ellershaw, J. and Wilkinson, S. (2003) *Care of the Dying: A Pathway to Excellence*. Oxford: Oxford University Press.

Gibbins, J., McCoubrie, R., Alexander, N., Kinzel C. and Forbes, K. (2009) 'Diagnosing dying in the acute hospital setting – are we too late?', *Clinical Medicine*, 9: 116–19.

Henwood, M. and Neuberger, J. (1999) *Debate of the Age Health and Care Study Group. The Future of Health and Care of Older People: The Best is Yet to Come*. London: Age Concern.

Irvine, C. and Devlin, K. (2009) 'Daughter claims father wrongly placed on controversial NHS end-of-life scheme', *The Daily Telegraph*, 8 September.

Jones, J. (2007) 'In search of a good death', *British Medical Journal*, 327(7408): 224.

Kraus, F. (2007) *Children, Young People and Loss*. London: St Christopher's Hospice.

Kyle, G. (2009) 'Terminal restlessness: causes, assessment and management', *End of Life Care* 3(3): 8–12.

Littlewood, C. and Johnson, M. (2006) 'Care of the patient dying from heart failure', Chapter 8 in M. Johnson and R. Lehman (eds), *Heart Failure and Palliative Care*. Oxford: Radcliff Publishing.

Marie Curie (2012) *Support for Children and Teenagers* [online]. Available at: www.mariecurie.org.uk/en-gb/patients-carers/for-carers/supporting-children/ [accessed 22 May 2012].

Milligan, S., McGill, M., Sweeney, P. and Malarkey, C. (2001) 'Oral care for people with advanced cancer: an evidence-based protocol', *International Journal of Palliative Nursing*, 7(9): 418–26.

Moyer, D. (2011) 'Terminal delirium in geriatric patients with cancer at end of life', *American Journal of Hospice and Palliative Medicine*, 28(1): 44–51.

National Cancer Institute (2010) *End-of-Life Care: Questions and Answers* [online]. Available at: www.cancer.gov [accessed 25 May 2012].

National Council for Palliative Care (2006) *Changing Gear: Guidelines for Managing the Last Days of Life in Adults*. London: NCPC.

National Council for Palliative Care (2007) *Artificial Nutrition and Hydration: Guidance in End of Life Care for Adults*. London: NCPC.

National Council for Palliative Care (2012) *Dying Matters: What Should You Tell Children about Death* (8th leaflet) [online]. Available at: www. dyingmatters.org [accessed 25 May 2012].

Rolls, L. (2008) 'Helping children and families facing bereavement in palliative care setting', in S. Payne, J. Seymour and C. Ingleton (eds), *Palliative Care Nursing*. Buckingham: Open University Press.

Step Mom (1998) Chris Columbus (Director). Columbia Pictures, USA.

Wee, B. and Hillier, R. (2008) 'Interventions for noisy breathing in patients near to death', *Cochrane Database Systems Review*, CD005177.

Worden, W. (2001) *Children and Grief* (2nd edn). New York: Guilford Press.

CHAPTER 9

Care after death

Joanna De Souza

This chapter will explore:

- What happens when the patient dies?
- Pronouncing the patient's death
- Supporting the relatives
- What happens if the family is not present?
- Care after death
- Being with a patient when they die
- Supporting my colleagues

Introduction

Being with someone at the point of their death can be the most wonderful and the most terrifying experience. Knowing what may happen and what to do can be helpful in relieving some of the anxiety at this time, both for you as a nurse but also for the family and friends who may want to be with the patient. This chapter will look at managing the last moments of life when the death is one that has been anticipated. By the end of the chapter you will have had an opportunity to reflect on what it may be like to be there when someone dies and have some idea of what needs to be done and what role you may play in that event.

Many people, when given the choice, choose to die at home. The following case study offers an opportunity to explore what procedures need to be followed at the time of death.

Dorothy and Bill

You are working in the community with a community staff nurse, Ola, and are going to visit Mrs Graham, who lives at home with her husband. She has end stage renal disease and her renal dialysis was stopped last week, after several years of treatment. Mr Graham called this morning and requested an early visit as he was concerned about his wife, whom you have come to know as Dorothy and Bill.

When you arrive at the house, Bill is very concerned and tearful. He expresses how Dorothy appears to be hardly breathing and at one time he thought she had gone, but then she breathed again.

When you go in Dorothy is looking very pale, she is only breathing occasionally and the breaths are very shallow. Her mouth looks dry and her eyes are closed.

You help Ola to moisten her mouth. Just as you are helping her with a small refreshing wash she lets out a small sigh and then she stops breathing. You call Bill back to her bedside and you all sit with her. She does not breathe again. After a few moments Ola gently asks Bill if she can check Dorothy's pulse and heart sounds. She does so and is able to say that Dorothy has died. Bill is very sad but it was a very peaceful end.

After some discussion, Ola phones Dorothy's GP who agrees to come to the house. Meanwhile you ensure that Dorothy looks comfortable and talk to Bill over a cup of tea. Bill has already received a leaflet from the hospice home care team called 'What to do when someone dies', so Ola uses this opportunity to talk through it with Bill and to discuss what he needs to do during the next few days.

What happens when the patient dies?

Degner et al.'s (1991) study looking at nurses' behaviours at the point of death identified seven key behaviours in nurses with palliative care expertise which are useful in helping us to understand what may be needed at this time:

- Responding to the death scene
- Providing comfort
- Responding to anger
- Enhancing personal growth
- Responding to colleagues
- Enhancing the quality of life
- Responding to the family (Degner et al. 1991)

Once it is suspected that the patient has died, it is important to complete some simple tests to ensure this is the case so that the family can be informed and you can help them to receive the news. The most appropriate person to do this depends very much on the situation in which the person has died.

To ascertain if someone is dead, listen to the heart for a heartbeat and feel for a pulse for one minute. Examine the patient's chest for any for signs of breathing, look at the patient's pupils to check pupil size and reaction to light.

When a person's heart stops and they stop breathing, the blood in their bodies will drain from the blood vessels in the top of their body down to the bottom, so after a short time, their upper body will appear pale, while their lower body may appear swollen or oedematous and dark. If the person is lying on their back, this may appear almost bruised.

Pronouncing the patient's death

The details of who can officially pronounce that someone has died were laid out quite clearly by the government in 2008 in *Confirming Death – Guidelines for Verifying Life Extinct* (DHSSPS 2008). They advised that this can be done by all doctors registered with the General Medical Council, and appropriately trained nurses and ambulance clinicians. 'Appropriately trained' usually means nurses who are working in a senior position in an area in which dealing with expected death is a regular part of their nursing role. For example, district nurses or nurses working in elderly or end-of-life specialist units.

Only registered doctors can sign the death certificate. However, in the case of the death being verified by another person, if the cause of death is easily evident, the doctor does not need to see the body to sign the certificate. If the patient has not been seen by a doctor within the last 28 days or is not thought to have died of natural causes, the case has to be referred to a Coroner's Court.

In the case of Dorothy, as you and Ola are the only health care professionals present in the house, it would be appropriate for Ola to make some general checks on Dorothy at this point. Although as a nurse Ola can make an initial assessment and suggest that Dorothy has died, it needs to be a medical doctor who fills in the death certificate that will be used by the family to register the death.

Supporting the relatives

Earlier in this book we looked at communication at the end of life (Chapter 3) and the role of the nurse, where possible, in offering families clues about the impending end of life. If they watch for these signs together, it is often a shared decision that the patient has died and, in this case, some deaths can be achieved quite peacefully. However, sometimes, even if the family is aware that someone is dying, they may not recognise that the patient has died or may be out of the room at that moment. Being able to share with the bereaved the details of the moments of death can be very useful in their grief journey. Much of the more recent bereavement literature (discussed in Chapter 11) describes the need of the bereaved to be able to understand and make sense of the death. It is often when this information is not available to them, or is unclear, that their anxiety is raised. Poor communication at the end of life between families and professionals is a very common source of hospital complaints as people can be left with many unanswered questions and their reaction to the loss and grief they are experiencing is to get angry and look for someone to blame (Kübler-Ross 1969).

Discussing the death when it may have been traumatic or distressing for the patient is particularly difficult and is explored more fully in the next chapter, which also looks at the situations where the death may have been sudden or unexpected.

In our scenario, Bill was an active member of the caring team right up to the point of death. Being there will have given him the opportunity to see what happened and to ask any questions he may have had at the time. Sometimes people have further questions later and good record-keeping by the health care staff involved can enable these to be managed well at a later date. If there are other members of the family nearby, you may have a conversation with Bill about whether they would want to come to the house before Dorothy is moved to the funeral directors. This experience may also allow an opportunity for them to ask any questions they may have.

What happens if the family is not present?

Families may not always be present at the time of death and it is important through forward planning and good documentation to know what is most important to them and how they would feel if they are not present for the death. When caring for someone who is very unwell, carers will often become exhausted and it is important to have conversations with them about their priorities and the need to also care for themselves. You may find some people are more concerned with being with the person and they express a wish that the patient is not alone. You can use this opportunity to discuss what you should do if they have gone home and the patient deteriorates. It is also important to offer a 'what if' scenario at this point.

> 'If something unexpected happens and 'X' deteriorates suddenly or dies unexpectedly, what would you want us to do and who would you want us to call first?'

Mentioning an impending death may be a difficult thing to do, but the clarity and honesty it gives to conversations and the plans people are making can be hugely beneficial. It changes the situation from an unexpected to an expected death and allows families to start the grieving process and prepare themselves. This information needs to be carefully and clearly documented so that the information is easily accessible when required.

Providing comfort

Being with a person and their family at the point of death can be a profound experience that may be intensely peaceful or very disturbing to those involved. The role of the nurse in this situation initially is to maintain calm (Degner et al. 1991). If family members are not present, then informing them and allowing them to be part of that time becomes a priority.

The more we understand and feel confident about what is happening and what needs to be done, the more we are able to offer that calming perspective. While it is important to be able to provide information about what to do next, being with a family who have just experienced a death can be a very special time, and we can enable that to be a positive rather than negative experience for people if we take the time to do so and fight the natural inclination to go into the information-giving role.

The moment someone dies can be very upsetting for members of the family, and it may be a time when a great deal of emotion is expressed. Learning to sit with someone while they cry, rather than feeling uncomfortable and trying to stop them, is a very useful skill in nursing.

Responding to anger

Not everyone will be just sad. Early bereavement work by Elizabeth Kübler-Ross (1969) illustrated that a common reaction to dying and death is anger. Where the loss is painful and perhaps associated with unresolved issues, the bereaved person can become very angry and distraught. Allowing people to vent their anger in a controlled way can offer them the opportunity to express the matters that are concerning them and to start processing for themselves what has happened. If you are faced with an angry relative, try to offer them an opportunity to talk but think about putting into place some of the communication strategies you have learnt in your training. This is further developed in Chapter 10.

Rituals and beliefs

It is also important to remember that some families or individuals may have special rituals that they will want to be performed after death. These may have religious, cultural or simply historical significance to the people involved. Open conversations prior to death with both patients and families can ensure that these are again documented in the patient's care plan and so can be facilitated by the professionals involved.

For example, Nyatanga (2008) refers to a Jewish custom of laying a feather over the mouth of the deceased for the first 10 minutes to ensure death has arrived and breathing has stopped. This may or may not be significant for a Jewish family in your care. I remember nursing a lady whose family was keen for her to be buried in her wedding dress, so we had to facilitate this being available so that we could dress her before it was difficult to put on such a tight-fitting garment. These days dressing patients once they have died is the role of the undertaker so those sorts of issues can be discussed at a later stage. However, immediate rituals can only be achieved if preparations have been made and discussions have been conducted early.

Walter (2003) and Vale Taylor (2009) have both undertaken studies looking at the importance of rituals and traditions in the management of the death scene and in the grieving process. They highlight some of the common rituals practised in the UK, predominantly those associated with families from a historically Christian background.

However, Vale Taylor uncovered that while families may be moving away from traditional church-based mourning rituals, they often create new and more individualised rituals during the mourning process, perhaps with the intent of maintaining some of bond with or memory of that person.

Looking at the literature, we see some common themes emerging from these rituals. They often involve some sort of gathering together of significant people, some sort of music or dance, often eating together – especially eating particular foods used in ceremonial gatherings – and perhaps some kind of tangible artefact. The universality of these types of ritual around the world shows our need, as social human beings, to connect with one another at these significant events.

Reflective questions

In your own family what happens when someone dies? What are the common practices and who does them? What role do other family members play?

What would you want to happen if someone close to you died? What role would you want to play?

Within your family situation, what might make this difficult for you?

Returning to our case study, Bill had lived in the area for many years and his family had always used a local firm of undertakers. While they were waiting for the doctor to arrive, Bill discussed what had happened at the funerals of his mother and his brother, both whom had died in the local area. He talked about how people gathered together for a service in the local church because although his family had not been regular churchgoers, they had celebrated their baptism, weddings and funerals in the village church. In addition, Dorothy had been an active member of a lunch club for older people that was run by the church for some years before she had had to stop when she started dialysis. He was sure the ladies from the club would provide the refreshments for the funeral as they had remained very supportive to Dorothy and Bill while she was unwell.

Perhaps not surprisingly, Bill and Dorothy had talked about the funeral arrangements and so Bill had already started to think about whom he would need to contact and what arrangements he would need to make.

Ola used the opportunity to go through the 'What to do when the patient dies' booklet that Bill had received from the community team. This contained the phone number of the local registry office where he would need to book an appointment to register Dorothy's death.

Once the doctor had visited and had had a cup of tea with Bill, you and Ola were able to help Bill lay Dorothy out and to ensure that she had on a clean white nightdress, at Bill's request.

Bill decided to wait until a little later before he called the funeral director as he was keen just to have a little more time with Dorothy before she left the house. Happy that he was OK, you and Ola left and were able to return to the community nurse base and pick up with some of your remaining workload for the day.

Facilitating different rituals at the point of death can be challenging within large institutions. Discussion with patients or relatives beforehand can allow you to plan with them and formulate an achievable plan. However, it is not always easy to achieve the environment and ritual that a family may want and as health care professionals we need to learn how to help families to manage those compromises at this difficult time.

Providing information

Another way to support families is to provide a variety of information leaflets, although it is not always easy to broach the subject or to pick the 'right time' to think about offering people information about what they will need to do after a death. So the information is often not given to the relatives until after the event has occurred, even if the dying person may have been known to be dying for a number of days.

At this stage the information can still work as a useful guide, although it is not able to serve the purpose of prompting discussion about future wants between either the patient or family or within the family. This is discussed in the previous chapter.

Reflective questions

Are there any information booklets available for the patients and carers in your area about what to do when someone dies? When are they given to relatives?

Are there other ways to make that information more accessible for the families you are involved with? This could be leaflets in outpatient and doctors' surgeries as well as on display in inpatient units, for instance.

How would you feel about giving such a leaflet to a family going through that watch-and-wait period that often occurs before someone dies?

Rehearse what you may want to say to them at that stage.

Care after death

The National End of Life Care Programme (NEoLCP) (2011) has produced national guidelines for managing the patient who has died and for conducting what has traditionally been known as 'last offices' or 'laying out'. They discuss a wish to move away from the term 'last offices' as it may hold militaristic or faith-based connotations for some people. They prefer the term 'care after death' as this can be seen as broader than the physical preparation of the body.

These national guidelines will be helpful in ensuring a practical and thoughtful approach to these important aspects of care. It is also important to be able to locate your hospital policy (which may still be called the 'last offices' policy), and to be familiar with it, as it will contain some detail about the specific location and people who you may need to involve in your Trust.

The national guidelines provide very specific detail about the way in which to prepare your patient after they have died, dependant on whether there is going be an inquest and referral to the coroner (discussed in the next chapter looking at unexpected death). They offer a rationale for the procedure and it is helpful to be familiar with this before you encounter the situation in your work. It will help you to avoid doing something that is inappropriate at the time, particularly in regard to removing IV lines, etc.

Some clinical areas or community teams have developed their own rituals around care after death. In hospitals where I have worked, the hospital mortuary has been renamed, for example, 'Rose Cottage', or people use euphemisms, such as 'He's going on a trip to the second floor'. These may or may not be helpful in terms of opening up conversations and ensuring clarity of understanding of the procedures necessary in the care after death. Other death rituals are explored by Walter (2003), including the laying of a flower on the pillow beside the deceased. Although the use of rituals in the process of grieving is very important, it is also important to clarify with the bereaved their personal wishes rather than to persist with traditional rituals that may cause distress.

Reflective questions

Have a look at the national guidelines (NEoLCP 2011) and reflect on your own experience of working with a patient who died. If you have not had this experience, perhaps you can look at it with a staff nurse colleague who has had that type of experience.

What aspects were known to you? What aspects were perhaps unexpected? Are there any local customs that would not fit with this protocol? Why have they come about? Do they need to be reviewed?

These days, much of the preparation of the body for cremation or burial is done by the funeral directors, and if family and friends are not present soon after death, it is recommended that they view the person who has died at the funeral directors' because bodies kept for any period of time without preparation in hospital mortuaries can present a distressing sight for the bereaved.

Whether or not it is important for people who have been bereaved to see the person after they have died, appears to be individual choice. Much work has been done in neonatal units on holding babies after they have died, which can become a very important and precious memory for that bereaved family. However, there has been some controversy after a NICE guideline was issued recommending that this practice was not routinely offered after some research showed that parents who do not hold stillbirth babies may in some cases recover sooner (NICE 2011). Nevertheless, current bereavement theory indicates that seeing the deceased helps with the process of accepting the reality of the death (Worden 2009).

If your place of work has booklets for people who are dying or for the recently bereaved, it is helpful if you can access these easily and quickly for the family, but they can also be a useful guide for yourself about what needs to be done. If you do not have an internal document, then have on hand some national leaflets from organisations such as Age UK, for example *When Someone Dies: A Step-by-Step Guide to What To Do* (2010). Another useful resource to offer families is the Home Office website, which provides detailed information about what is required to register a death following certification. It is helpful if hospitals and community teams individualise this information into Trust-wide leaflets as they can then contain quite specific information such as the address and contact details of local registry offices.

Being with a patient when they die

Anxiety about what the needs of that patient may be just before death and whether they are in distress is often a worry for people caring for the dying, especially if it is for the first time. Fear that the patient may die unattended, either by you or by the relatives, for whom the vigil is important, is another worry that is commonly held.

When death is expected and symptoms such as terminal restlessness (discussed in previous chapter) are managed, death often comes almost unnoticeably. If the patient has had breathing difficulties, death can be signified by a sudden quietness that can, at times, feel eerie. Alternatively, as people are often in quite a sedative state prior to expected death, the change is almost imperceptible and it is only when you notice they have become fixed in expression or become very pale that you notice they have died.

Being prepared for the death experience and being open as to how it may affect you is a good place to be when it happens. Getting on with your case load after an experience such as being with Dorothy while she died can, on the one hand, be disturbing and somehow feel disloyal to her memory; however it can also be an uplifting experience as you feel like you have been part of a very significant part of someone's life. There are a number of nursing poetry sites on the internet and many of the poems focus on an experience of being with a dying person. It shows us how significant such events can be.

Confidence and experience always feel like the next step of the journey but how do you get there and learn what to say when you are just starting out? Having the opportunity to observe another competent member of staff dealing with death can be helpful as you can see how they manage the situations and questions that arise. However, being with a senior member of staff who deals with death very differently and incongruently from your own culture of behaviour may be a challenging situation to deal with. The use of reflection can be very helpful in that circumstance.

Degner et al. (1991) discuss how some nurses develop a role for themselves that involves enhancing the death experience for patients and so develop the ability to feel at ease when a patient is dying and to utilise their knowledge in the area to enhance their nursing care. The study compares this with the experience of nurses who feel anxious about dealing with death, and have a sense of regret if the outcome for a patient is death. They found a sense of enhanced growth in those who were able to see this as role development.

Supporting my colleagues

Respecting each other's individual rituals and beliefs around death is particularly important. Some staff may not have had much experience of patients dying, or a particular death may have affected them profoundly. Being aware of the emotion involved in such an event, anticipating it and being able to share with another person the significance of the event to you is an important aspect of supporting colleagues. Being prepared to listen but also to share your own feelings and interactions can provide both team members with some support.

Doka (1989) discusses the notion of disenfranchised grief, which is a common feature in large institutions where death may happen relatively often and there is a need to move on and, for example, utilise the bed space for another patient. However, how does this feel for the colleague who is not on duty on the day or at the time when the patient died? Do we have any kind of systems in place to recognise the relationship that has been lost and allow for that member of staff to hear the narrative of the death and therefore start to make sense of it for them? This will be covered in more detail in Chapter 12.

Summary

The key points to remember when considering caring for someone after they have died are:

- There are a number of physical signs that can give us an indication of when a patient is coming near to the very end of life.
- A clearly designated person will need to verify death when it occurs.

- Highlighting to friends and family that someone has died is more difficult if they have not been present for the death. Thinking about what you may say beforehand can be useful preparation.
- Anger is a natural reaction to loss, particularly through death. Allowing people to express their anger in a controlled environment without becoming defensive can allow people to start to explore what has happened to them.
- Each Trust has a 'last offices' policy. Care needs to be taken to explore with friends and family what death rituals may be important to them so that you can try to facilitate them for the family.
- Peaceful death can be almost an unnoticed event. Spending time caring for someone who has died allows us to offer them dignity which can be helpful in managing our own sadness.

Further reading

Read the National End of Life Care Programme and National Nurse Consultant Group (Palliative Care) (2011) guidance for staff responsible for care after death: National End of Life Care Programme and National Nurse Consultant Group (Palliative Care) (2011) *Guidance for Staff Responsible for Care after Death*. London: DH. This helps us to prepare for how we might care for people after they have died in a sensitive and appropriate way.

Julia Lawton's work, looking at the experiences of people who are dying and the experience of those that care for them, is a very interesting if sometimes slightly disturbing account that may be useful when preparing relatives for what can sometimes be a long drawn out process of dying: Lawton, J. (2000) *The Dying Process: Patients' Experiences of Palliative Care*. London: Psychology Press.

References

Age UK (2010) *When Someone Dies: A Step-by-Step Guide to What To Do* [online]. Available at: www.ageuk.org.uk/money-matters/legal-issues/what-to-do-when-someone-dies/ [accessed 25 May 2012].

Degner, L.F., Gow, C.M. and Thompson, L.A. (1991) 'Critical nursing behaviours in the care of the dying', *Cancer Nursing*, 14(5): 246–53.

DHSSPS (Department of Health, Social Services and Public Safety) (2008) *Confirming Death – Guidelines for Verifying Life Extinct* [online]. Available at: www.dhsspsni.gov.uk [accessed 25 May 2012].

Doka, K.J. (ed.) (1989) *Disenfranchised Grief: Recognizing Hidden Sorrow*. Lexington, MA: Lexington Books.

Kübler-Ross, E. (1969) *On Death and Dying*. New York: Routledge.

National End of Life Care Programme and National Nurse Consultant Group (Palliative Care) (2011) *Guidance for Staff Responsible for Care after Death*. London: DH. [See Further reading]

NICE (National Institute for Clinical Excellence) (2011) *Review of Clinical Guideline (CG45): Antenatal and Postnatal Mental Health – Clinical Management and Service Guidance.* London: NICE.

Nyatanga, B. (2008) *Why Is It So Difficult to Die?* (2nd edn). London: Quay Books.

Vale Taylor, P. (2009) 'We will remember them: a mixed-method study to explore which post-funeral remembrance activities are most significant and important to bereaved people living with loss, and why those particular activities are chosen', *Palliative Medicine,* 23: 537.

Walter, T. (2003) 'Hospices and rituals after death: a survey of British hospice chaplains', *International Journal of Palliative Nursing,* 9(2) 80–5.

Worden, J.W. (2009) *Grief Counselling and Grief Therapy: A Handbook for the Mental Health Practitioner* (4th edn). New York: Springer.

CHAPTER 10

Sudden or unexpected death

Joanna De Souza

This chapter will explore:

- What makes sudden death traumatic for the patient?
- Management of end-of-life care emergencies
- Communication – the forgotten palliative care emergency?
- What makes sudden death traumatic for you as a professional?
- Dealing with unexpected death
- What makes sudden death traumatic for the family?
- Caring for the relatives after the death
- Other issues that arise with unexpected death

Introduction

Interestingly, when you ask well people how they would like to die, many talk about dying quickly or in their sleep, as the idea of a lingering death is an uncomfortable one. However, in reality death that comes suddenly and unexpectedly can be very difficult for both the patient and, in particular, for those left behind, even for the more experienced staff. It can be a traumatic and tiring experience for yourselves as a team and you may often also be dealing with traumatised relatives or friends. If there are no supporters, this in itself can make this situation difficult and stressful. This chapter will look at some of the issues that arise and at some of the ways we can try to work in these situations to reduce the anxiety and trauma of all involved.

The following case study illustrates a position that we can find ourselves in both in hospital or in the community. Sometimes we have not been working with the patient long and haven't really had a chance to develop a relationship with them. This case study highlights some of the initial challenges, particularly around communication.

Bupa

You are on a night shift on the intensive care unit (ITU) and you are looking after Mr Patel, whom you know as Bupa, who came into hospital with a high temperature and feeling very unwell about a week ago. Bupa has had cancer of the colon for three years and is now having palliative chemotherapy for lymph and lung secondaries. He was diagnosed with neutropenic sepsis and has been on a range of different antibiotics and IV fluids. A discussion has been held with Bupa and his wife, Asmeeta, and it has been decided that should Bupa have a heart attack (arrest) he will not receive cardio-pulmonary resuscitation (CPR). However, Bupa and his family are keen to continue with other active supportive care interventions to manage his infection.

Asmeeta and Bupa's mother, Mrs Patel, have been sitting with him much of the time but were exhausted and went home late last night to get some rest. Bupa has a daughter who has been supporting her mother and a son who lives in Sydney and is flying home. He is due to arrive tomorrow afternoon to see his father.

At handover, the evening staff nurse expressed concern about Bupa. He remains very hot and his temperature is above 38 degrees. His breathing is becoming laboured and they are worried he is developing a chest infection. His blood pressure is high despite a variety of medications. He is very clammy to touch and his hands are cold and cyanosed. He is difficult to rouse but has been so for a couple of days. The staff nurse reported that the doctors are aware that he does not appear to be responding to the antibiotics. They are planning to have a discussion with the oncologist and then with the family the next day once Bupa's son has arrived.

Overnight you notice that Bupa's breathing becomes shallower and his pulse becomes weaker. Over the next hour Bupa's blood pressure drops and his breathing becomes quite difficult. The registrar on call discusses the situation with the ITU consultant and they do not feel that it is appropriate to put Bupa on a ventilator. As a team, you decide to administer more IV fluids, but he continues to deteriorate. A busy half an hour later, Bupa dies.

What makes sudden death traumatic for the patient?

Sudden deaths take on many forms. In the past we would often talk about people dying 'at home in their sleep'. There are a number of conditions where people are at risk of dying as they sleep, such as sleep apnoea (where a person's homeostatic mechanisms do not promote reflex breathing while sleeping), or people may fit, suffer unexpected heart attacks (myocardial infarctions) or strokes (cerebral vascular accidents) and die very quickly before anyone else is aware they are unwell. The condition 'sudden infant death' is one where this may happen with a child.

It is obviously very difficult to know how this feels for the patient and although some have facial expressions that indicate they may have suffered discomfort at the end, it is not really possible to determine the extent and duration of that distress or pain. For many patients that we work with as health care professionals, sudden death is often preceded by a period of intense illness which can be uncomfortable, traumatic and undignified for patients. Many patients who do die unexpectedly in health care settings, such as in the case of Bupa, are often acutely unwell beforehand and may have a high burden of symptoms and medical interventions taking place. Some of these will be potential causes of discomfort, such as high fevers, symptoms of nausea, catheters, intravenous infusions, etc.

Being aware that death is imminent allows for anticipatory grieving, where patients can use the time before an expected death to sort out their affairs and to engage in ending rituals with others that can be helpful (Reynolds and Botha 2006). However, for many, the unknown quality of their final hours causes some anxiety and, for some, a real fear.

End-of-life care emergencies

Sadly, unexpected death may often be associated with severe and uncontrollable symptoms or life events that make the whole situation difficult for everyone. Television dramas often display sudden deaths brought about by trauma, either in combat or through accidental death situations. In most cases the deaths are swift and involve only momentary suffering for the person dying. In reality this is rarely the case.

Some situations we may meet when working with people at the end of life that may result in death are referred to as palliative care emergencies. High blood calcium levels (hypercalceimia) and spinal cord compression have been covered in Chapter 7 and breathlessness, including stridor, in Chapter 8. In a sudden death situation other distressing emergencies may include haemorrhage, seizures or sepsis. The palliative care team in Lothian and Lanarkshire (NHS Lothian 2010) have produced some helpful guidelines in dealing with some of these.

Haemorrhage

Being present when someone has a haemorrhage can be very distressing. Occasionally someone may have an internal haemorrhage where there may be no obvious sign of a bleed; the patient may suddenly become sleepy, very pale (cyanosis) and then drop into a coma. If the bleed occurs within the abdomen, there may be no external signs that it is a bleed. However, realising that someone has just suddenly died like that can be quite a shock.

If the bleed occurs within the gastrointestinal tract, the cyanosis may be accompanied by vomiting blood (haemoptysis) or bloody diarrhoea (malaena). This can be very distressing for all involved and health care professionals need to act quickly to take command of the situation. The first step would be to call for assistance – you are going to need others around to help. If possible, obtain dark coloured bed clothes, dressing gown or towels to mop up the blood. Look for the origin of the bleed and if possible apply pressure to the area to stem the blood flow until more help arrives. If you are able to stem the blood flow, the patient may enter cardiac arrest but be in a position to require resuscitation, so this would need to be commenced. If the bleed is internal or uncontrollable, the patient may well be agitated by the event and rapid sedation may be given. In this situation it is likely that the patient will lose consciousness relatively quickly.

If there is any indication that a patient is at risk of having a catastrophic bleed, a preparatory plan and conversation, particularly with relatives, is really important. It may allow you to have suitable equipment and medications at hand (for example, at home) and to alert staff to the possibility of it happening so that they move quickly when it occurs. Decisions about resuscitation can also be clearly understood by all involved as it is difficult in situations like these emergencies to check all the required documentation if these factors are unknown. Families can also be prepared about what actions they can take in this very difficult situation.

However, it is important to recognise that no amount of preparation can take away the trauma of being present at such an event and opportunities to talk about it and to work through our emotions and fears afterwards are really important.

Seizures

Seizures or fits can occur in patients who have raised intracranial pressure due to trauma, tumours or electrolyte imbalances. Again, often there are cues in a patient's condition that allow professionals in non-emergency situations to be able to identify when a patient is at risk of seizures and we can start to have preparatory conversations with patients and families about what actions they might need to take should one occur. Although this may be a difficult and upsetting conversation to have, it can allow the event to be a little less traumatising for the patient and carer if it does occur.

If your patient does start to fit, if possible place them in a recovery position to increase the chances of helping them to maintain an open airway. If the fitting is severe and prolonged, anxiolytics can be used. If prepared, relatives at home can be involved in this administration.

Familiarisation of the local Trust policy on the management of seizures can be helpful in understanding the more extended aspects of care and implications this may have for the patients involved.

Sepsis

Sepsis can be described as the body's reaction to infection (Surviving Sepsis Campaign 2012). Severe sepsis is one of the leading causes of death as it results in the interruption to the blood supply of major tissues and organs. Often, the immune system of patients who already have an existing life-threatening illness is impaired so they are at an increased risk of sepsis due to a lack of neutrophils (the main white blood cells involved in fighting infections). In this situation, people are described as being in neutropenic sepsis. This lack of first-line defence against infection means that treatment needs to be given quickly and at appropriate doses in order to be effective.

Early recognition of infection and risk status is very important and again patient and carer education is important. Decision-making around treatment options for sepsis is also important. The Surviving Sepsis website can be a useful resource for exploring many of these issues.

Bupa and his family had considered what they would want done should Bupa develop an infection and as a result he was treated with intravenous antibiotics. However, his situation was complicated by their decision for Bupa not to be resuscitated in the event of cardiac arrest. It is important for the team in intensive care to revise this situation with Bupa and his family so the whole team is clear on the priorities of care. These can be difficult times and patients and families may choose to make changes to decisions they have made previously. Our role as health care professionals is to be able to support them to do this, but I feel it is equally important to be able to support them to stay with the decisions they have made previously when not under the emotional strain of the current situation.

Communication – the forgotten palliative care emergency?

Pickering and George (2007), two palliative care physicians, ask this question in a thought-provoking piece in the *British Medical Journal*. Using an increasingly common example of a patient with heart failure who is fitted with an implantable resuscitation device, they explore the importance of initiating conversations to reduce the incidence of sudden, unexpected and, as a result, traumatic death situations simply because of a lack of communication and discussing those difficult topics before they arise.

Worden (2009) also discusses the importance of giving understandable information about potential dangers and ensuring we do not conceal the risks of treatment that people undertake. He encourages engagement with expressions of grief and other painful emotions in the face of the crisis of illness. Perhaps it is in fear of this that we, as health care professionals, do not engage in the level of discussion we need to with patients and families facing life-threatening decisions.

What makes sudden death traumatic for you as a professional?

As professionals, we see ourselves as the people who should be in control and also as the people who should know what is happening. Therefore we feel we should be able to manage our patients through the situations in which they find themselves when they come into our care. Dealing with unexpected events is something we learn to manage as we progress on our learning journey. However, some unexpected events remain stressful, often due to their far-reaching implications, and sudden death is often one of these.

This is well captured by Saines (1997) in her phenomenological study of the experiences of qualified nurses dealing with sudden death situations in accident and emergency (A&E) departments. A&E departments do not always see themselves as providers of end-of-life care but the first categories that emerged from the stories that were told by these nurses were how often they encounter death in their work. These deaths were nearly always in situations where they were sudden and unexpected for all concerned and not knowing the patient and family only created additional stresses.

The nurses in Saines' study discussed the stress of facing a situation in which it becomes obvious the patient is going to die. They recalled the difficulties in dealing with their own reactions to this loss of life and also that of often very distressed relatives. The last concept that arose from the study was the pain of reflecting on these situations because their suddenness and unpredictability often means that there are elements of unresolved business connected with them.

Sometimes when patients die on an inpatient ward, following a period of illness, they have (over time) become stripped of their individuality. Often they wear hospital night clothes if they have required many changes. Sometimes their families or friends are not present for much of the time, as social contact is controlled by ward visiting policies. We as nurses may be keen to keep a sense of tidiness and order. Lawton (2000) offers an interesting discourse around this concept. How much does this socialisation reduce the individuality of the situation and thus reduce one source of potential stress for the health care professionals caring for them?

Having some relationship with our patient, Bupa, and his wife and family allows us to be able to consider what may be a suitable approach for this particular family, and when we make the phone call to tell the family about Bupa's death.

For student nurses there may be added elements that make the situation difficult. In her study, Loftus (1998) looked specifically at the experience of student nurses, for whom dealing with people who were dying was still a relatively new experience. She found that student nurses found it very stressful when patients suddenly deteriorated and died. On exploration, she found that they felt that often the qualified staff seemed to beware at an earlier stage than the students that the patient wasn't going to recover, as they had seen and recognised warning signs that the students had missed. Sometimes it appears that when acquired knowledge becomes so intuitive, we forget how much we draw upon subtle cues that may not be obvious to all. As a result, students often found themselves in the situation of dealing with sudden deterioration but without appropriate support from their more senior counterparts.

Reflective questions

Can you recall a situation in clinical practice where someone deteriorated much more suddenly than you had expected?

Looking back, what were the signs that the person was becoming more unwell? How did you manage your emotions around that situation?

Dealing with unexpected death

Caring for dying patients in a very technical situation was a second theme that arose from Loftus's work as a stressful situation for students (Loftus 1998). This is shared by qualified nurses (Saines 1997).

One of the most stressful situations students found themselves in were unsuccessful cardiac arrest situations. Much of this anxiety centred on feelings of helplessness and incompetence. However, some anxiety was also experienced due to the feelings of the inappropriateness of the cardiac arrest procedure with patients who were known to be terminally ill. This stress is played out graphically and beautifully in the film *Wit* (2001), in a complex scene where a primary nurse has engaged in a difficult but very rewarding conversation with a patient about their final wishes which are then over-ruled by another member of staff with the result of a very undignified death.

Reflective questions

Wit, starring Emma Thompson, is an American film detailing a woman's experience of cancer. If you can, watch the film and, in particular, reflect on the Popsicles scene and the one which follows it. The situation in the film has perhaps been exaggerated for its impact factor, but it highlights some pertinent issues.

The first scene shows a nurse discussing bad news, and concentrates on making the decisions about whether or not to resuscitate and how the nurse handles both her own and her patient's emotions on this subject. The following scene is more traumatic as the patient's final wishes are disregarded. Reflect on how this made you feel.

Thinking of patients you have looked after who are near the end of their lives, who makes the decisions about resuscitation? Do you think that some patients may opt not to be resuscitated if given the choice?

The nurses in Saines' (1997) study felt particularly distressed by the memories that will be left with families following a sudden and traumatic death:

> It bothers me that people will just remember the feeling in the resuscitation room as their last memories of their loved one. (Saines 1997: 168)

It can leave worries about our own competencies in dealing with the situations in which we find ourselves. Jezuit (2000) explored the suffering that nurses experience when working with people at the end of life and challenges the management to ensure that there are appropriate systems in place to support them. One such intervention is the opportunity to formally reflect on a stressful situation such as a sudden death which allows the nurse to identify what actions were taken and the appropriateness of them. If this can be done as a team, this often provides an opportunity for validation of actions and affirmation that, given the circumstances at the time, the actions taken were appropriate. It also allows all professionals involved an opportunity to understand the whole event. This can be extremely helpful in future interactions with bereaved families and provides huge opportunities for developing more effective ways of working and future strategies for such situations.

Most Trusts will have a local policy for managing after-death care and most of these will have a section for unexpected death situations. It is important to be familiar with these guidelines and to refer to them when the situation arises to ensure that we do not do things that we should not have done.

What makes sudden death traumatic for the family?

Worden (2009), a grief psychotherapist, in his work looking at the grieving process, discussed what he called *mediators of mourning*. These are the factors that may affect how a person responds to a loss such as death. They are the things that can make experiencing the loss easier or harder for that person. One of these mediators is how the person died. How the death occurs can make quite a difference to how it affects the bereaved person.

Anticipatory grieving or prior warning is known to be helpful in allowing people facing a loss to start experiencing the pain and to begin adjusting to the realisation of the impending loss. However, when the death is sudden, the bereaved are *robbed of this preparatory grief* (Worden 2009). It can also be more difficult to accept the reality of the loss, particularly when you may not have seen any sign of deterioration. When people die in settings like intensive care units, sometimes the opposite may occur, where the relatives assume things must be getting better as the person who was very unwell and perhaps in obvious distress seems to be breathing well and appears calm due to ventilation and sedation.

Part of the anticipatory grieving process is the provision of an opportunity to tie up loose ends. People can use this time to begin to resolve any issues they may have in regard to the loss. Some people use this time to undergo a process of bargaining (Kübler-Ross 1969), where they look to other avenues than the ones tried to prevent the loss from occurring, such as trying new treatments or diets, etc. In a sudden death situation, there is not time for any of this type of work and the bereaved can be left feeling guilty for not having tried different avenues or for not having resolved outstanding issues. In a complicated situation like suicide or accidental death, the bereaved can be left feeling responsible for the death because they may feel they did not do enough to prevent it.

Upon realising that the death has now occurred and cannot be reversed, people are often overwhelmed by a feeling of helplessness. Parkes and Prigerson (2010), in their theory of loss, talk of the feelings of numbness that can follow any type of loss. However, in sudden death this is amplified by the unpredictability and unreality of the situation. There is an immediate loss of control over life events. A common reaction to this is a feeling of frustration and anger that exhibits itself as *a need to blame*. Neimeyer and Anderson (2002), in their model of narrative reconstruction, discuss the need of the bereaved to try to make sense of their loss and what has happened to them. When the loss is very sudden, people seek desperately for there to be concrete reasons for why the death occurred and therefore look for someone to have made an error which caused this unexpected outcome. Their displaced anger and this need to find an obvious reason for the death will often result in confrontation between health care professionals who may have been involved in the care of the deceased and the family, particularly when the full information around the circumstances of the death are either unknown or unavailable to the bereaved.

The sudden nature of unexpected death often leaves many questions and a gap in information. Bearing in mind the emotional state of the newly bereaved, initially people find it very difficult to take in and understand what has happened, if they are told quite soon after the death has occurred. Sadly, sometimes information given at this time is limited by the health care professionals because they are also keen to find meaning in a death situation before they engage in much information-giving to families. They need to ensure that there were no avoidable errors and they need to consider if there is any culpability for poor practice.

This can be difficult within health care teams where different members of the team feel differently about what information should be given, how it should be done and to whom. Settings in which death occurs more frequently often have established policies and patterns for handling information-giving and communication with the bereaved. Hospices often have very established follow-up sessions, such as day after death meetings, six week follow-up and a further follow-up available for complicated bereavements.

Interestingly, settings such as intensive care units, which are also centres that experience high volumes of complicated dying situations, seem less prepared for this.

Caring for the relatives after the death

Asmeeta

After some discussion between yourself, your mentor and the registrar, it was decided that Asmeeta should be called in to discuss the situation. As your mentor knew Asmeeta best, she said that she would call her at home and explain that Bupa had deteriorated suddenly in the night and had died, and ask her to come in.

The phone call was a difficult one and Asmeeta was very upset. However, she, her mother and her daughter decided to come up to the hospital as soon as they could. Your mentor asked you to stay near the nursing station so that you could speak with them as they arrived on the ward and before they came to Bupa's room, while she worked with the registrar with Bupa. Your biggest concern was what you would say to Asmeeta.

One of the other common models used for the breaking bad news is the SPIKES model, formulated by Robert Buckman (2005). Buckman is a medical doctor who has written extensively about communication, particularly in connection with difficult conversations. Although Buckman's model is primarily designed for medical staff preparing for a pre-planned consultation, it still offers us a useful framework for situations such as preparing to speak with Asmeeta.

S – **SETTING**

P – **PERCEPTION**

I – **INVITATION**

K – **KNOWLEDGE**

E – **EMPATHY**

S – **S**TRATEGY and **S**UMMARY

S – Setting

If possible, and it may be that you only have a short time, thinking through and preparing for an event such as breaking bad news is invaluable. It allows you to enter the situation with a plan rather than just a reactive approach.

Think about location. Where would be a good place to take the relatives when they arrive to have the conversation? It needs to be somewhere you can sit down and speak privately. Alert your colleagues to your plan and minimize interruptions.

You may initiate your discussion, perhaps directing it first to Asmeeta, but include the others:

> *Nurse*: Asmeeta, I am so sorry, thank you for getting here so soon. Please come and sit down so that we can discuss exactly what has happened.

P – Perception

Buckman (2005) suggests that we start the interview with an evaluation of the bereaved person's perception of the events so far. Asking people to tell their story provides a number of useful elements in this situation. It allows them to take some control in a situation in which they have begun to feel so out of control. It also allows us as the professionals to ascertain their level of understanding of what has happened. We also know from the bereavement work of writers such as Neimeyer and Anderson (2002) that there is a therapeutic value in people telling their story as they seek to find meaning in what has happened to them.

> *Nurse*: Asmeeta, I think Sarah rang you at home, didn't she? Can you tell me what she said to you on the phone?

I – Invitation

Perhaps in this situation it may seem obvious that the bereaved person will want to talk to you about what has happened. However, some people may be so distressed or be carrying with them such a burden of anger or other emotions, they may not wish to talk at this stage. Buckman (2005) highlights the importance of looking for an invitation from the other person and to use this as your cue for further intervention. Again, this allows the bereaved person to have an element of control in the situation.

> As Asmeeta starts to explain what happened, she stops talking, weeping quietly. None of the others says anything; they too are weeping. You wait with them for a few moments and offer round a box of tissues from the table nearby. After what seems like a long and slightly uncomfortable silence, Asmeeta, continues in a quiet voice. ...

K – Knowledge

This is a suggestion to consider both the knowledge held by the bereaved person but also the knowledge they may require and the sort of language that may be the most helpful for them.

It is important to value and acknowledge the death by using clear terminology. We are often tempted to soften the news with the use of terms such as 'he is no longer with us', 'he has gone to a better place', or 'he has passed away'. In situations of unexpected death, and particularly when the bereaved have not been present for the death, it is important to be clear to help them to accept the reality of the death.

Worden (2009) suggests that it is important to have established, as part of your preparation for this meeting, exactly what happened as far as possible, as people are often seeking correct information that is given with a sense of authority. In sudden death situations, the bereaved often have an increased need to understand the precise nature of the death and what happened. We see this played out on our television screens with highly publicised inquests, such as the *Marchioness* disaster on the river Thames, the Potters Bar rail crash and following the London bombings. Although it is very painful for the bereaved, they are often quoted as gaining relief from knowing exactly what happened and are more able to begin the process of working through their grief once the facts are known.

Take time to give the precise details as far as you are able. It is also important to consider the language you will use in this situation. We need to ensure that there is clear understanding, although it is also helpful to use some of the medical terms that the bereaved person may read on death certificates or other information pertaining to the person's death and to clarify understanding of these. If possible, it is good to try to make this a discussion rather than a one-sided conversation as responses can often indicate where there are misunderstandings or the particular aspects that are distressing.

Nurse: Asmeeta, can you remember how Bupa was when you left this evening and what was happening with him?

Asmeeta: When we left he was fine, just sleeping.

Nurse: That's right. We had just given him his evening antibiotics and although his temperature was high and his blood pressure was still high, his breathing seemed stable. You sat with him for so long, you know he was.

After you left, the evening nurses continued to watch him and as you know we were trying to balance his blood pressure while also giving him enough fluid and antibiotics to try to take control of the infection.

When we came on, we took the report and did his observations. Poor Bupa was quite sweaty so we gave him a little wash down and he did look more comfortable. However, when Sarah and I went to do his antibiotics and observations at 12:00, he had become more pale and his blood pressure had fallen down.

Asmeeta: Yes, Bupa's blood pressure was usually around 130/65.

Nurse: Because of his temperature, we were keen to try to give him some more fluid so we immediately called Alex, the doctor, to come and reassess him and in the mean-time again sponged him down to try and make him more comfortable. Alex came up quite quickly as he was only on the ward next door and he increased the rate of fluids. Then, Asmeeta, it happened so fast, Bupa's breathing became really shallow and he just deteriorated and then he stopped breathing. We had discussed whether we should call the crash team, but we had discussed this with the two of you, if you remember, and it had been decided if it got to that stage, it may not be the best thing for Bupa to go through cardiac resuscitation as he was so vulnerable [...].

I am so sorry there was not time to call you. Asmeeta, for himself, he was peaceful and he had a dignified death. He did not appear to be particularly conscious of any suffering at the end. We were with him, and we thought of you and your family.

E – Empathy

Sometimes people may respond in very unexpected ways. There may be anger, there may be laughter, there may be hysterical crying. One of the challenges of working with bereaved people is the unpredictability of emotional response to loss. Allowing expression of loss is helpful and being able to offer any clarification that is required may also be helpful.

Silence is also good. It allows space for this discussion to sink in and for Asmeeta to raise a response, which may be in the form of a question or just an expression of sadness.

S – Strategy and summary

Worden (2009) discusses the importance of helping people to actualise the loss. In sudden and unexpected death situations, seeing the deceased can also help the process of accepting the reality of the death. This may be particularly helpful with children who at younger ages are very concrete thinkers. Viewing the body can also provide an opportunity to involve the bereaved in helping to prepare the body for removal to the funeral directors. For many, this final care-giving can be a precious way of feeling involved with this stage of life, especially if they were not able to be there at the death.

As you come towards the end of your conversation with Asmeeta, it may be helpful to offer support in thinking about the next stage after she has been to see Bupa. It may be at that stage you offer her some advice about what procedures need to be done next. It may be helpful to have obtained beforehand a hospital leaflet that will outline the procedures in that particular setting. It is useful to establish for yourself where these are kept, what is in them and how to access new supplies when those on the ward run low.

The needs of the bereaved can be broken down into their needs directly after the death and their needs in the longer term. The former is considered in more detail in Chapter 9 and the latter is covered in more detail in Chapter 11.

Other issues that arise with unexpected death

Following any kind of unexpected death, there may be additional factors to be considered. It is important for all involved to be clear about the cause of death, so when this is not clear there is often a requirement to involve a coroner.

Coroners and inquests

A coroner is an independent judicial officer, who must be either a lawyer or a doctor, and is sometimes both. They are paid by the local authority and they oversee an inquiry into sudden deaths where the cause is unknown, or into deaths where there may be an indication of unlawful activity. The Ministry of Justice (2010) has produced a useful leaflet which outlines the role of the coroner and when they would need to be involved in a case.

Often with a hospital death, the coroner will use the documentation available, including the patient's notes, and nursing staff or family members do not need to be involved. However, the family may have to wait for the coroner's outcome before they can have the funeral. If it is a more complex case, there may need to be more involvement by family or staff with the investigation, particularly where there may be issues of intentional harm or neglect of duty. It is useful, as professionals, for us to be aware of these to be able to guide and prepare family and friends.

Organ donation

Organ donation is a difficult subject in health care. On the one hand, organ transplant teams lose up to a third of their patients because they die before an organ becomes available. In acute care settings, health care staff feel unable to burden grieving families with decisions about organ donation. Campaigns have been run as to whether we should move to an opt-out system, where it is presumed that people want to donate their organs unless they carry a card or have used some other means to demonstrate they would prefer not to have their organs removed. However, there have been many objections on religious and moral grounds, so we continue with the opt-in system.

Much has been done to improve people's awareness of donation issues and most hospitals with a trauma centre have an organ transplant team who offer an on-call service to come and speak with relatives if there is any possibility of organs becoming available for transplant.

Action point

Explore how to contact the organ donation team in your place of work. Can you arrange to spend a day with them, or attend a session on organ transplant issues in your Trust, or visit the team and find out a little more about how they work and when it would be most appropriate to involve them in your area?

Religious and cultural issues

When the death is unexpected, often communication around death rituals needs to be done retrospectively, but it is important to enable death rituals to be put in place where feasible as soon after the death event as possible. If a coroner does need to be involved, this may prevent some of these rituals, such as being buried before sundown on the day of death, so it is important to acknowledge how difficult this may be for a family and how it may add to the grief of their bereavement.

The sudden death of a child

Cook, White and Ross-Russell (2002), three paediatricians, recognised that it can be particularly difficult when dealing with the sudden death of a child. They offer a model based on their experience of dealing with families in this situation. The model is based on the need for a bereavement follow-up meeting, which is standard practice in paediatric care and perhaps should be so in all areas of care.

They suggest that formal clinician-led meetings should not be held immediately but should be scheduled a short period after the death, that is 8–12 weeks later. This meeting will then allow for any new information surrounding the death of the child to be clarified so that answers can be given. The meeting should be structured initially to allow the concerns of the family to be raised. Wright (1999) emphasises the importance of using this opportunity to give people chance to tell their story. Wright found that the process of reliving the events of the day of the death is integral to enabling the bereaved to process their experience. This discussion also allows for clarification of any ongoing misunderstandings.

Following this, support issues, such as sibling support, should be discussed and professional assistance should be offered. For some families, revisiting the ward or place of death can be helpful so this should also be offered. Lastly, at least one of the professionals conducting the meeting should be aware of the signs of pathological grief so that this can be followed up if necessary.

Reflective questions

Are follow-up clinician-led meetings part of the routine care offered to patients dying in your setting? What role can nurses play in being part of this?

Would you be supported in changing a shift or in coming into work outside your normal working hours to enable such a meeting to take place in your setting?

Would this be a helpful process for you too in ending what may have been a traumatic event for yourself?

Looking after ourselves

Sudden death can also be traumatic for the health care professionals involved and may result in a number of unanswered questions for the team. As the work of Loftus (1998) and Saines (1997) illustrates, it is helpful to be able to debrief and reflect on what has happened to allow both qualified and unqualified staff an opportunity to think through their experience, understand what happened and perhaps to offer new insights for future care.

For Bupa's family, and particularly for his son who sadly arrived after his father had died, having a good relationship with the health care team who had cared for Bupa, and being able to have open conversations about what had transpired, will help all the family to start to work through what has happened to them and the loss that they have experienced. Not being present for the death can be a complicating feature for all the family as they face bereavement. However, being able to now engage in mourning rituals that are important to them may give them some space and time before they have to fully engage with the pain of their loss.

In addition, your role in supporting them to have been involved in the decision making about what treatment Bupa would want and being able to offer a sensitive approach to information giving may really help them on their journey to accepting some of the unpredictability and inevitability of his death.

Summary

The key points to remember when considering the care required by patients and families facing sudden or unexpected death are:

- Sudden death is made more complicated when it is completely unexpected. Sometimes deaths are more unexpected for relatives than they are for us as health care professionals because we refrain from alerting them to the cues that we have to identify when someone's health is deteriorating.
- Sudden death can result in complicating factors such as relatives not being present at the death and the need for medico-legal authorities to become involved.
- Involving family members and being clear in communicating with them about what has happened helps to alleviate some of the anger and confusion that often accompany grief reactions.
- Sudden death can also be traumatic for health care professionals and debriefing is a helpful tool for them too

Further reading

William Worden is a psychologist who has co-ordinated post-traumatic stress support in a number of different situations, particularly in the aftermath of the 9/11 bombings. His work offers a useful insight into the grieving process that occurs following death, especially those that are sudden or unexpected: Worden, J.W. (2009) *Grief Counselling and Grief Therapy: A Handbook for the Mental Health Practitioner*. London: Routledge.

References

Buckman, R.A. (2005) 'Breaking bad news: the SPIKE strategy', *Community Oncology*, 2(2): 138–42.

Cook, P., White, D.K. and Ross-Russell, R.I. (2002) 'Bereavement support following sudden and unexpected death: guidelines for care', *Archives of Disease in Childhood*, 87: 36–9.

Jezuit, D.L. (2000) 'Suffering of critical care nurses with end-of-life decisions', *MEDSURG Nursing*, 9: 145–52.

Kübler-Ross, E. (1969) *On Death and Dying*. New York and London: Routledge.

Lawton, J. (2000) *The Dying Process: Patients' Experiences of Palliative Care*. London: Routledge.

Loftus, L. (1998) 'Student nurses' lived experience of the sudden death of their patients', *Journal of Advanced Nursing*, 27: 641–8.

Ministry of Justice (2010) *A Guide to Coroners and Inquests* [online]. Available at: www.direct.gov.uk [accessed 25 May 2012].

Neimeyer, R. and Anderson, A. (2002) 'Meaning reconstruction theory', pp. 45–64 in N. Thompson (ed.), *Loss and Grief*. Basingstoke: Palgrave.

NHS Lothian (2010) *Palliative Care Guidelines: Emergencies in Palliative Care (Version 2)* [online]. Available at: www.palliativecareguidelines.scot.nhs.uk/symptom_control/emergencies.asp [accessed 25 May 2012].

Parkes, C.M. and Prigerson, H. (2010) *Bereavement: Studies of Grief in Adult Life* (4th edn). London: Psychology Press.

Pickering, M. and George, R. (2007) 'Communication: the forgotten palliative care emergency?', *British Medical Journal*, 334(7606): 1274.

Reynolds, L. and Botha, D. (2006) 'Anticipatory grief: its nature, impact, and reasons for contradictory findings', *Counselling, Psychotherapy and Health*, 2(2): 15–26.

Saines, J. (1997) 'Phenomenon of sudden death', *Accident and Emergency Nursing*, 5(4): 205–9.

Surviving Sepsis Campaign (2012) Society of Critical Care Medicine [online] www.survivingsepsis.org/Pages/default.aspx (accessed 18 February 2012)

Wit (2001) Written by Emma Thompson and Audra McDonald. Directed by Mike Nichols. London: CineScene.

Worden, J.W. (2009) *Grief Counselling and Grief Therapy: A Handbook for the Mental Health Practitioner*. London: Routledge.

Wright, B. (1999) *Sudden Death: A Research Base for Practice*. Edinburgh: Churchill Livingstone.

CHAPTER 11

Supporting family and friends

Joanna De Souza

This chapter will explore:

- Understanding the landscape of loss
- Theories and models of loss
- Supporting patients who are facing loss
- The end stage of grieving
- Other ways of considering the grieving process
- Supporting families who are facing loss
- Mediators of mourning
- Your empathy and emotions

Introduction

Working in health care involves meeting people facing loss on a daily basis. Any kind of ill health is associated with losses. However, when working with patients and their families facing life-limiting illness (and particularly when approaching the end of life), we often become more acutely aware of the very specific losses they are facing. How can we help them through this very difficult time?

The End of Life Care Strategy (Department of Health 2008) outlines the importance of care after death as the sixth step of the pathway. How the NHS should be providing this care is laid out in the National End of Life Care Programme (2011) document, *When a Patient Dies*. Its main aim is to encourage the use of a bereavement pathway which highlights the important elements of bereavement care required. Some of the aspects are covered in previous chapters of this book, and how we understand and prepare our patients and families for the time after death is the focus of this chapter.

Lydia Jones

You have been allocated to look after Lydia Jones, a 73 year-old, who is very unwell and in the process of dying. She has a syringe driver in place containing antiemetics, pain relief and some sedation as she has been having problems with a number of symptoms, including haemoptysis (vomiting blood).

Lydia lost her husband 10 years ago as a result of a heart attack. She has two children who have families of their own. Ron, Lydia's husband, had worked for the diplomatic service and as a result they had lived abroad much of their lives. While abroad, Lydia contracted hepatitis C following a blood transfusion after a road traffic accident, for which she received some treatment with interferon.

Over the past three years Lydia has become increasingly tired and has developed symptoms of liver disease, such as nausea, abdominal pain and yellowing of her skin and the whites of her eyes (jaundice). The team did discuss the possibility of a liver transplant, but Lydia, after careful consideration, decided she did not want to go through that level of treatment.

Lydia was admitted through A&E following an episode of haemoptysis (vomiting blood). Her youngest daughter, Chloe, lives locally and has been visiting her mother daily while she has been in hospital. Her children are at secondary school and manage to get to and from school without their mother. Her ex-partner lives nearby and has shared custody of the children. Lydia's oldest child, Eleanor, lives three hours' drive away but has young children who are at primary school, so although Eleanor came over for the first couple of days after her mum was admitted, it is not easy for her to stay for long. You are anxious that you may be looking after Lydia when she dies and are not sure what you will say to the family or how it may be best to help them when the time comes.

Understanding the landscape of loss

Facing loss is often a constant part of the experience of families and carers of people with life-threatening illness. Machin (2009) uses the helpful analogy of the 'landscape of loss' to illustrate the multitude of losses that often accompany ill health.

First, there is the loss of control and 'normality' when serious illness comes into the family. It brings much uncertainty, loss of understanding of what the future holds and often higher demands on time and resources so other elements of normal living may need to be compromised. Roles may need to change and along with all of this may come the pain of knowing you are losing someone who is valuable to you.

Reflective question

What kinds of losses do you think will be experienced by Lydia and her family?

Lydia has had a loss of health which will have changed her whole way of life and ability to function as she did before. This is often associated with a loss of independence and choice. She will also have experienced a loss of control over what her future will hold with the diagnosis of her hepatitis C infection. Alongside her health losses, she has lost her husband. He died unexpectedly from a heart attack, so his death may have resulted in a number of changes for Lydia, including perhaps where she lived. As Lydia's health deteriorates, she may have to face more physical losses as she becomes less able to look after herself and perhaps increasingly reliant on assistance from others to carry out her daily care needs and in meeting her health care needs. Depending on the skills of her carers, she may also lose dignity if she becomes excluded from the decision-making process of her care.

Lydia's children have experienced the loss of their father and then now the knowledge that they will slowly be losing their mother. Chloe may experience losses associated with daily life and being able to care for her children; Eleanor, possibly faces losses associated with not being able to share precious time with her mother. As we grow older and our parents grow older too, often the roles change and this can result in losses of security and provision where we may become the provider and have to take on new responsibilities. The partners of Lydia's children may be experiencing losses associated with Lydia's decline, depending on the relationship they have built up with her. Lydia's grandchildren will also be affected, and there may be some friends that play a significant role in Lydia's life who may also be experiencing loss.

Doka (1989, 1999) developed the theme of disenfranchised grief. Disenfranchised grief refers to losses that people have that aren't always acknowledged or validated or recognised by others. He warns that someone who is isolated in bereavement may find it more difficult to mourn and their reactions may often be complicated. Ex-partners, such as Chloe's, hidden relationships, children and grandchildren often fall into this category.

Understanding ourselves

Before we look at how our patients and their families react to loss, as health care professionals, we need to gain insight into our own experiences of loss and our reactions to it. Knowing about the processes and reactions of people facing loss and knowing some practical strategies will help us to judge what to say when working with bereaved families (Brown and Farley 2007). This will enable a more insightful understanding of some of the behaviours we may observe in the families we are working with.

First, it is helpful to look at what we mean by some of the terms frequently used when thinking about loss. In Worden's (2009) book on grief therapy, he begins by looking at the terms 'grief', 'mourning' and 'bereavement'. He describes grief as the experience of the loss, whereas Doka (1999) describes it as the reaction to loss. Mourning is described by Doka, amongst others, as the process one goes through to adapt to the loss, and bereavement defines the loss one is trying to adapt to.

Reflective questions

Think about a loss you have experienced of something that was significant to you. It does not need to be someone who has died.

Think about your reaction when you first discovered or knew of the loss. Record how it felt, how it affected your thoughts, and how you behaved at the time and just afterwards. How did these reactions change over time? How do you feel about the thing that you lost now?

Keeping these reflections in mind, we will explore some of the literature on bereavement, grief and the process of mourning.

Theories and models of loss

Early grief observations were made by Sigmund Freud, who in his work *Mourning and Melancholia* (1917) discussed the concept of 'grief work', which he saw as a thinking (cognitive) process people had to go through to work through their loss. He observed that in general people seemed to go through this process and reach an acceptance of their loss in order to move on and start new relationships. Much of his work as a psychoanalyst, seeing people with problems, seemed to relate to where people had not been able to complete this 'grief work', but had become stuck in the process and unable to detach from the person who had died. It remains common today that a significant number of people seeking psychiatric help have an unresolved grief reaction (Worden 2009).

In 1944, Lindemann conducted some research looking at the responses of people bereaved through a factory explosion. He captured the array of behaviours and emotions he found in the people he was working with. He found that there were similar patterns in the behaviour of the recently bereaved: bodily distress of some kind, preoccupation with the image of the deceased, guilt relating to the deceased or the circumstances of the death, hostile reactions and an inability to function as competently as they did prior to the death.

Reflective question

Thinking back to the last reflective question, how did your thoughts, feelings and behaviours reflect those you see in your patients or carers who are experiencing loss?

Worden (2009) explores some of these reactions when he looks at the behaviours of the bereaved today. We see people in that initial reaction after hearing or realising their loss become numb, unable to concentrate, often breaking down and perhaps remaining very tearful. Think of patients following the news of a new significant diagnosis. Often they are unable to remember what the doctor has said except for some things that have really registered for them, like the word cancer or a prognostic time.

Sometimes in the newly bereaved we see some of those behaviours identified by Lindemann (1944): searching, trying to play the event over and change it, anger, sometimes looking for someone to blame to give the loss some kind of meaning. In public displays of grief we often see shrines, songs created, pictures and lots of activity around the image of the deceased.

Lindemann also found some similarities in the process people seemed to go through following the loss event:

- Accepting the loss as a definite fact
- Adjusting to life without the deceased
- Forming new relationships in the world.

Further exploration of these then led to the development of theories and models that can be used by practitioners to understand what people may be going through and, in particular, to be able to identify what is normal grief and what is abnormal grief that may need some specialist intervention.

Bowlby's (1982) work on attachment found – through studies looking at the attachment process that occurs between infant and mother – that separation resulted in a loss reaction which caused the reactions of grief documented in the literature. This breaking of these bonds of attachment account for much of the grief reactions we see and provided a basis for much of the work on loss reactions.

Sometimes diagnosis with a life-threatening illness challenges those attachment bonds and we see families reacting in different ways. Perhaps, like Lydia's daughter Chloe, a vigil develops, where family members will want to spend considerably more time with the person they may be about to lose. Sometimes this can be overpowering for the ill person and it can lead to family tensions, particularly where patients wish to retain their autonomy but grief reactions in other family members result in over-protectiveness.

Concern about the way dying people were treated by the medical profession in America in the 1960s led psychiatrist Elizabeth Kübler-Ross to look further into this area. Her seminal work in 1969 was a study of the experience of people facing death. This study demonstrated many behaviours similar to those identified by theorists such as Lindemann, in those being bereaved. It led to an understanding that we see grief behaviours in people facing death as well as in those grieving for one who has died. Since then, further work has demonstrated that grief behaviours are reactions to many types of loss, not just those involving death (Harris 2011). Kübler-Ross went on to develop a model based on her studies and observations.

From theories to models

You might perhaps be familiar with Kübler-Ross's stage model. She describes five stages that people pass through as they 'come to terms with' their loss. The stages are: (1) shock and disbelief, (2) denial that the loss event has happened, (3) anger that may be fuelled by guilt that more could have been done, (4) fear or anxiety of what this may mean, and finally (5) acceptance that the loss has occurred, but that a sense of peace about it has been achieved, and an ability to move on.

This work has played a transforming role in the recognition that the process of experiencing loss is complex and that some of the behaviours we see in people experiencing loss may be about their own thought processes about the loss rather than really being directed against those around them, as they may appear. Murray Parkes, a palliative care consultant at St Christopher's Hospice in South London, through his extensive work with the dying and the bereaved, developed Kübler-Ross's work to produce a model that was a little less prescriptive. Rather than stages, it centres on phases that people go through, such as numbness and despair to acceptance (Parkes 2001).

Disadvantages of stage models

Although Kübler-Ross did not intend her work to be used prescriptively, and only in a linear fashion, many practitioners working in the field using these models have been found to be applying them in that way. Professionals, seeing certain behaviours, are keen to categorise and often pathologise them, for example, 'she is in denial', or 'she is stuck in anger', as if it were a negative process. This can result in professionals not taking active steps to explore what the issues are in these situations and assuming that over time these people will simply move on to the next stage. Other professionals working with loss have found that the passive nature of the models does not really reflect what they see.

Worden's task model

Worden (2009), through his work as a psychologist working with bereaved people, developed the idea of a model based on tasks. He saw the process as a much more active one than the passive processes described by Kübler-Ross and Parkes, interestingly returning to Freud's notion of grief work.

Worden's four tasks involve:

- Task I: To accept the reality of the loss.
- Task II: To process the pain of grief.
- Task III: To adjust to a world without the deceased.
- Task IV: To emotionally relocate the deceased and move on with life.

His model postulates that people actively engage with processes such as experiencing the pain of loss, in some way perhaps to move through the phases offered by Parkes.

Supporting patients who are facing loss

So what about our patient Lydia? How might we apply this understanding of the grieving process to working with her and helping her with her bereavement? Worden's task model allows us to see how we might start to understand the process she may go through.

Task I: To accept the reality of the loss

Other chapters have focused on the importance of early discussions and their role in giving people time to adjust to their loss and to perhaps resolve some life issues and be involved in future care decisions. During this time we may also be able to offer Lydia opportunities to talk about how she is finding things and what is happening to her, allowing her opportunities to find meaning in her experiences of loss of her health, roles and ability to fulfil the plans she may have made for her life.

Task II: To process the pain of grief

This is often one of the hardest tasks. Loss is almost inevitably linked with sadness of some type as those attachment bonds are broken. We find it hard to allow our patients to experience pain, particularly psychological pain, and often we feel tempted to either avoid it by not raising difficult subjects or by trying to make them feel better with reassurance.

Reflective questions

Think about the last time you were with a patient or a relative who was crying. How did it make you feel? What did you feel you should do?

Learning to sit and share a patient's pain by being with and listening and talking about difficult things, without dismissing it with an 'Oh, don't worry I am sure it is going to be OK!' is a valuable skill that comes with practice and reflection.

Task III: To adjust to a world without the deceased

What a challenge, to move to a place where immortality becomes less of a priority than making the most of the time that is left. Kübler-Ross, in her model, talks of a time of acceptance that perhaps for many was not so much acceptance but the beginning of the process of detachment. Families often really struggle with patients when they enter this stage, and we hear them say 'She is giving up hope...', as explored in Chapter 7. What is hope in end-of-life care is another interesting concept which is touched up in Chapter 1.

Task IV: To emotionally relocate the deceased and move on with life

Perhaps Lydia will not complete this task. Julia Lawton (2000) conducted a study looking at patients in hospices and she documented what she called the dying process. She identified some patients who appeared to become emotionally detached and ready to move on. In some of the work looking at the frail elderly, we sometimes see some of this occurring. Perhaps we may instead see Lydia maximising her time with her children and particularly her grandchildren as she develops Klass, Silverman and Nickman's (1996) continuing bonds.

The end stage of grieving

Another far-reaching change that began to occur in the loss literature was a move from a final stage of acceptance and somehow replacing and moving on from the loss object, to a relocating of the emotional energy connected with the lost object (person), retaining some kind of ongoing but perhaps different relationship with them. Worden (2009) changed his last task from letting go of emotional attachments to the deceased and allowing them to invest in the present and the future, to finding an enduring connection with the deceased in the midst of embarking on a new life. However, whether there is an end stage to grieving, or whether we always retain a place for the lost, is a question asked by some contemporary theorists.

Klass, Silverman and Nickman's (1996) work on continuing bonds explored this concept and developed a new type of theory that looked at how, as people moved on through life following loss, they maintained rather than severed the bonds with the deceased.

Other ways of considering the grieving process

Some recent theorists have moved away from the idea of these more prescriptive models and particularly the notion of grief work as a sense of active, ongoing and effortful work. They recognise that grief is highly individual and that individuals grieve in their own way (Doka 1989), so the process may be more dynamic and long term than has been previously suggested. Examples of newer theories and models include Stroebe and Schut's (1999) oscillating model of restorative grief and the notion that it might not be phase-related or about grief work at all, and Walter's (1996) and Neimeyer and Anderson's (2002) work indicating that grieving may be more about finding meaning in the events that have happened to us.

In their extensive writing, Margaret Stroebe, her husband, William Stroebe and their collegue, Helmut Schut (1999) struggled with the grief work hypothesis that dominated the grief literature at the time. Instead, they developed their dual process model (Stroebe and Schut, 1999). This is based around an ideology that people facing loss are exposed to two types of stressor. Stressors that are loss-oriented, focus on the emotions and experiences of what has been lost and the grief that is associated with it. This may involve a preoccupation with a recently-deceased family member and displaying behaviours identified previously as searching or blaming, and so on. Stressors that are restoration-oriented, on the other hand, focus on events to do with ongoing life and the need to adapt to new challenges, often because one's social situation has changed as a result of the loss. These may include things like suddenly have to learn to operate all the gadgets in the house that previously their now deceased spouse used to operate (see Figure 11.1).

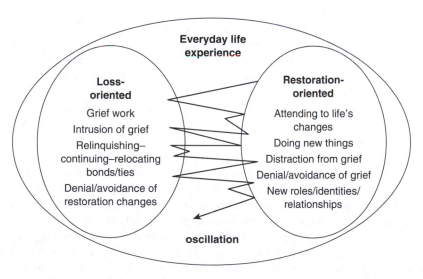

Figure 11.1 Stroebe and Schut 1999

Stroebe and Schut (1999) propose that people can at times confront and at times avoid the stressors in either orientation and so oscillate from thoughts that are concentrated on the loss object to thoughts that focus on what is happening to them now and are not connected to their loss.

Perhaps this is what we see sometimes when we use the term 'denial', and perhaps it also explains why sometimes people can lose themselves in something and almost forget for a short time the pain and grief of their loss (we see this at funeral wakes when the presence of extended family and friends can result in much enjoyment and merriment).

This process of oscillation is how we manage to survive the pain of loss but also manage to reintegrate back into life as we grieve. Stroebe and Schut (1999) suggest that close to a loss experience, people will often remain mainly in the loss orientation but over time may spend more and more time in reality orientation. However, over time, particular events or significant dates or memories may result in a person oscillating from reality orientation to loss orientation some significant time after the loss has occurred and perhaps retain the ability to do this forever. When we see our grandmother weep on her dead husband's birthday many years after his death, has she not got over her grief, or is she simply oscillating briefly back into a loss orientation and feeling the sadness she did at the time of his death?

This oscillation may result in the experience of quite intense emotions similar to the emotion they may have felt at the time of their original loss. Personal experience of this has been as a result of seeing a photograph or remembering a time spent with a lost loved one.

Finding meaning

Theories such as those offered by Walter (1999) and Neimeyer and Anderson (2002) see grieving and mourning as a process of 'healing grief' where, through creating a narrative, telling and retelling of our life stories or loss experiences, we go through a process of meaning reconstruction. This is a process of finding new meanings to reaffirm and rebuild our life in a world without the thing we have lost.

Like Lindemann (1944) and Worden (2009), we see an initial preoccupation with the loss. You have perhaps experienced this where the grieving person tells you the same story time and time again, and for a while you feel they may be 'losing their mind' as they don't seem to realise they have told you before. Neimeyer and Anderson (2002) would argue that this is part of the healing grief. That each time the person retells their story they reframe it in their own minds, and you become really a sounding board. This process allows them to gather more meaning each time they tell their story, and to make more sense of what has happened to them.

In my practice as a community palliative care nurse, understanding this was a revelation moment for me. I would often say 'Oh, don't worry, so and so has told me what happened', as someone started to retell me their story, hoping to spare them their distress, but in actual fact I realised I was denying them the opportunity to narratively reconstruct. Much traditional bereavement counselling involves offering people the opportunity to narratively reconstruct over a period of time until they reach a stage when they can cope with the pain of that grief.

Supporting families who are facing loss

So how can we use this knowledge and understanding to help us in our work in supporting families experiencing loss, particularly through end-of-life issues?

Using the dual process model

Let's think about Chloe and Eleanor first. Stroebe and Schult (1999) propose that when first exposed to a loss, people find themselves centred in loss orientation. There is often a period of intense anxiety and the family often gathers together and almost take residence with each other. This could be before or after Lydia's death and it may occur more than once as different losses are faced. During this time we may see a number of loss behaviours, as described by Lindemann, though in the midst of this we also see both Chloe and Eleanor spend some time in reality orientation while they deal with the realities of family life. They may also spend time in reality orientation making sense of the new relationship they will now have together, one in which there will not be a parental role player.

Sometimes family members can feel guilty or judge others who seem to be able to oscillate into reality orientation more easily than another. There is sometimes an expectation that all will grieve in a similar manner and within the same time frame. When this differs for individuals it causes concern and anxiety for others affected by loss, who often gain reassurance from shared experiences of grief with others feeling the same as themselves. Being able to both give people time to talk about their worries in this situation, but also to help them understand that the oscillating process is normal, can be reassuring for people and avoid judgements of insufficient grieving or people being in 'denial'.

Knowing that the pain of loss can be a long-term process and that we in fact perhaps always maintain a bond with the deceased is also useful for people to understand, so there isn't concern about 'not getting over' a death. However, it is important to be aware of risk factors that do make people more vulnerable to pathological and prolonged grieving. Worden (2009) describes these as mediators of mourning.

Mediators of mourning

Many current theorists would suggest that although grieving, particularly following a significant loss, is a sad and difficult experience, most people are able to engage in the process and find some way to reintegrate into normal life. However, the mediators of mourning can offer an indication of where the grieving process may be more complex, and when people may need some extra support in their grieving process.

Some of these mediators include who the patient was and the nature of the attachment to that person. If the attachment has not been secure, this may complicate the grieving process. This may sometimes be the case if there has been a family conflict at some point in the past.

A second mediator may be the mode of death and circumstances around it, particularly if the death was sudden or unexpected or in some way complicated. This was discussed in Chapter 10. In most hospices and in many community services, health care professionals will make contact or arrange an appointment to see the bereaved on the day after death. This is usually a meeting designed to clarify what happened and to offer an opportunity for the bereaved to tell the story of their experience. It allows the health care professionals to clarify any misunderstandings and answer any questions they may have at the time. In acute Trusts this meeting will often be held with the bereavement officer of the Trust. While they may take care to ensure they have the correct details about what has occurred, in general they can often only answer very general queries and if further clarification is required, a formal meeting needs to be arranged, often with the clinician in charge of the patient's overall care. This lack of ability to clarify minor details with people who were present, or who had obtained details directly from someone present, is perhaps one of the reasons so many complaints about NHS care focus around patient deaths and difficulties of communication.

Action Point

Establishing a good relationship with Chloe and Eleanor while you are caring for Lydia, and ensuring you take time to talk to them about what is happening, may really help with this final need for understanding.

How the death fits with the normal course of life is also a mediator. Thus, young deaths or any situations when a child dies before a parent, even if the child is an adult, are often complicated. Previous losses may also become a mediator if they have been complicated or recent. In addition, ongoing issues may also become a mediator if these are in themselves stressful. For Chloe and Eleanor, there may still be some issues around how their mother contracted the hepatitis C that eventually led to her death. Again, allowing for discussion and exploration of these if they emerge as an issue is important, even though it may feel that it was some time ago. Sometimes families harbour strong resentments against GPs who they feel did not refer the patient soon enough for treatment. Some of this may be part of the 'need to blame' element of grieving and in time they may resolve this for themselves.

However, sometimes they need to take action to be able to process the emotions they have around that event.

Being aware of these mediators of mourning are helpful in identifying with family and friends who may be at particular risk during bereavement. The National End of Life Care Programme (2011) encourages all clinical areas to develop a bereavement pathway that will steer all staff through this process and offers guidelines about who to contact if risk factors become evident through the period of a patient's care.

Your empathy and emotions

Understanding our own losses and how this has affected us is important in developing empathy and also in understanding our own emotions when faced with the loss of others.

Understanding theories such as Stroebe and Schut's dual process model (1999) can be helpful in understanding why, when we recall a significant loss that happened some time ago, we may suddenly feel quite an intense sense of emotion. This appears to be very normal and is not an indication that we have not 'got over our loss'. We may also hold a special place in our lives for the thing that was lost. The idea that acceptance and moving on from the loss, or even replacing the lost object (Bowlby 1982), certainly does not occur in many situations.

Understanding our own values and beliefs (Brown and Farley 2007) is also really important. Particularly important is the awareness that these have arisen through our upbringing, and a particular family or cultural background may be quite different from that of others.

Summary

The key points to remember when considering the experience of our patients and their families when facing loss and bereavement are that it is important to:

- Understand the family, the relationships within it and some of the loss-related behaviours we may see exhibited by them.
- Foster open communication between all family members, but also give opportunities for individuals to have a professional listening space for their own experiences and needs.
- Be able to offer family members some understanding of the processes they may be going through and that of others so that they can be able to support each other more effectively.
- Ensure clear and open communication between families, patients and health care professionals to allow for clearing up of miscomprehensions and clarification of any anxieties people may have due to a lack of knowledge or understanding about what is or has happened to the person at their death.

Further reading

Having developed a general understanding of bereavement, it is interesting to explore the work of Strobe and Schut and their oscillating model: Stroebe, M. and Schut, H. (1999) 'The dual process model of coping with bereavement: rationale and description', *Death Studies*, 23(30): 197–224.

Daryl Harris, working with Robert Neimeyer, offers a really interesting exploration of people's experience of loss where it is wider than loss through death. This is referred to as non-finite loss. Their book helps us to explore all the losses our patients may be facing and how this understanding may help us care for them:

There are several films that look at people coming to terms with the loss of a loved one, for example:
Stand By Me (1986) Ron Reiner (Director). Columbia Pictures: USA.
Steel Magnolias (1989) Herbert Ross (Director). Tristar Pictures: USA.
Eye For an Eye (1996) John Schlesinger (Director). Paramount Pictures: USA.
Pay It Forward (2000) Mimi Leder (Director). Warner Bros Pictures.

References

Bowlby, J. (1982) *Attachment and Loss. Vol. 1: Attachment* (2nd edition). New York: Basic Books.
Brown, J. and Farley, G. (2007) 'Supporting the family facing loss and grief', Chapter 9 in S. Kinghorn and S. Gaines (eds), *Palliative Nursing*. Edinburgh: Churchill-Livingstone.
Department of Health (2008) *The End of Life Care Strategy*. London: DH.
Doka, K.J. (ed.) (1989) 'Disenfranchised Grief', in *Disenfranchised Grief: Recognizing Hidden Sorrow*. Lexington, MA: Lexington Books.
Doka, K.J. (1999) *Disenfranchised Grief: New Directions, Challenges and Strategies for Practice*. USA: Research Press.
Freud, S. (1917). *Mourning and Melancholia*. The Standard Edition of the Complete Psychological Works of Sigmund Freud, Volume XIV (1914–1916): On the History of the Psycho-Analytic Movement, Papers on Metapsychology and Other Works, 237–258 [online] www.barondecharlus.com/uploads/2/7/8/8/2788245/freud_-_mourning_and_melancholia.pdf (accessed 17 June 2012).
Harris, D (2011) *Counting Our Losses: Reflecting on Change, Loss, and Transition in Everyday Life* (Series in *Death, Dying and Bereavement*, Edited by R. Neimeyer). New York: Routledge.
Klass, D., Silverman, P. and Nickman, S. (1996) *Continuing Bonds: New Understandings of Grief*. USA: Taylor & Francis.
Kübler-Ross, E. (1969) *On Death and Dying*. New York and London: Routledge.
Lawton, J. (2000) *The Dying Process: Patients' Experiences of Palliative Care*. Place: Psychology Press.
Lindemann, E. (1944) 'Symptomatology and management of acute grief', *American Journal of Psychiatry*, 101: 141–8.
Machin, L. (2009) *Working With Loss and Grief: A New Model for Practitioners*. Sage Publishers. London
National End of Life Care Programme (NEoLCP) (2011) '*When a Person Dies': The Guidance for Professionals on Developing Bereavement Services*. London: NHS.

Neimeyer, R. (ed.) (2001) *Meaning Reconstruction and the Experience of Loss*. Washington, DC: American Physiological Association.

Neimeyer, R. and Anderson, A. (2002) 'Meaning reconstruction theory', pp. 45–64 in N. Thompson (ed.), *Loss and Grief*. Basingstoke: Palgrave.

Parkes, C.M. (2001) *Bereavement: Studies of Grief in Adult Life* (3rd edn). London: Routledge.

Stroebe, M. and Schut, H. (1999) 'The dual process model of coping with bereavement: rationale and description', *Death Studies*, 23(30): 197–224.

Walter, T. (1996) 'A new model of grief: bereavement and biography', *Mortality*, 1(1): 7–25.

Worden, J.W. (2009) *Grief Counselling and Grief Therapy: A Handbook for the Mental Health Practitioner* (4th edn). New York: Springer.

CHAPTER 12

Resolving my own feelings after a patient has died

Annie Pettifer

This chapter will explore:

- What motivates health professionals to care?
- How I might be affected when a patient has died
- How registered practitioners might be affected by patients' deaths
- The sources of support that are available
- Burnout
- Developing resilience

Introduction

Although trained for a particular job, health care professionals are also individual people with their own unique background, current situation, personality and values. Inevitably, when faced with sad situations health care professionals may be personally affected in some way. Sometimes this is transitory and manageable; at other times it can be profound and overwhelming, even to the point of obstructing their ability to care for other patients or enjoy life beyond work. This chapter will focus on finding positive ways of coping with difficult feelings when caring for dying patients by following the case of Peter. Peter is a student nurse who returns to work following a long weekend off to find that, sadly, Mark, a patient with whom he has formed a close bond, has died. While this case follows one scenario, it raises a whole spectrum of questions about the nature of professional caring and appropriate relationships within it. This chapter aims to develop your awareness of these issues as a professional carer, and thereby equip you to care for yourself better when faced with difficult feelings.

Peter

CASE STUDY

Peter is a second-year student nurse aged 42. He married in his late twenties but sadly his wife died of breast cancer some seven years ago. They did not have children. He is a keen motorcyclist and both he and his girlfriend Gemma are active in his local club. After college, Peter gained a job with a local accountancy firm with which he was able to study and qualify as an accountant. However, as the years passed Peter felt less and less fulfilled with this role and decided to re-train as a nurse, hoping it would be both more interesting and more fulfilling.

His placement in a rehabilitation hospital had been positive. From the outset Peter felt welcome, and his mentor has spent some time with him explaining the model of care offered in the hospital. Peter found that watching people improve a little each day was rewarding. Many of the patients had had a neurological trauma, such as head injury, and had been referred from acute hospitals for a period of intensive rehabilitation to maximise their function. They would often be discharged with appropriate care in the community and, if needed, ongoing outpatient rehabilitation.

By the middle of his placement Peter had forged good relationships with the patients but he particularly enjoyed nursing Mark, a 59 year-old family man having rehabilitation for a intracranial injury following a road traffic accident while he was riding his Yamaha. The accident left Mark with limited co-ordination (ataxia) and visual disturbance, coupled with limitations to his cognition. Mark seemed to enjoy company and both Mark and his family seemed to appreciate someone who shared their passion for motorbikes.

When Peter left for his long weekend off he left Mark jovial and pleased with the progress he had made, but when Peter returned to the ward sadly he found that Mark had died during the previous night from an intracranial hematoma. Peter felt hugely saddened by this and he remained low for the rest of the placement. Although he was polite to the patients, he just did not want to get to know them well. He mentioned his feelings briefly to his mentor, but she seemed unaffected, saying that patients dying was simply something you have to get used to. Peter wondered whether in fact accountancy would have been an easier career choice.

Peter's situation illustrates the dilemma that many health care professionals face. We often choose caring professions because we enjoy caring for others and like the sense of 'doing something worthwhile' that it brings. Much of this job satisfaction stems from engaging meaningfully with patients and their families as individuals. However, in doing so, we can become vulnerable to a plethora of emotions, including experiencing sadness and loss ourselves. These can be particularly intense when we get to know several patients and families undergoing profound loss over periods of time, or when we are going through difficult periods in our own lives and with our own families.

Reflective question

Have you had a similar experience to Peter? You may wish to reflect on how you respond or might respond when someone you have particularly enjoyed caring for has died or faced profound loss. Have you ever been concerned about the way you have been or will be affected?

What motivates health professionals to care?

Perhaps the best place to start exploring what motivates health professionals to care is to consider the nature of caring itself. Understanding the nature of caring and our attraction to it can illuminate our motivation to care and what we gain from engaging in professional caring relationships. Developing such awareness is key to understanding why we may experience strong emotions when caring for people who die.

Many prospective students, eager to be accepted on health care training programmes, say that they are caring people or enjoy caring for others, and that this quality has motivated them to study to become a health care professional. However, they often find it difficult to put into words what caring specifically is and why it is so important to them.

Kirby (2003) offers us the following definition of caring. This suggests that the desire to care for others is a deep-seated, fundamental human drive to behave in a way that enhances the lives of others:

> Caring is more than having concern or being concerned for others, it entails commitment – reaching (out) to others intending to care. Care emerges from a deep moral source within; from a primordial concern for others we are compelled to act.
> (Kirby 2003: 24)

> ## Reflective question
>
> Cast your mind back to your decision to study to be a health care professional. What attracted you to caring?

Using Kirby's definition, people who choose to care professionally may strongly identify with this desire within themselves, and seek, through education and training, to develop their skills and ability to care effectively in a professional context.

Research corroborates the significance of caring in the motivation of nurses. For example, Newton et al. (2009) interviewed Australian undergraduate student nurses, registered nurses, nursing managers and directors about their motivation to choose and stay in nursing. Common to all groups was the desire to help others, caring and having a sense of achievement. It seems that knowing that we have helped others in some way, whether big or small, can hugely increase our sense of our own worth and self-esteem. This is particularly evident when our efforts are demonstrably appreciated by patients and their families. In short, caring for others can make us feel good about ourselves and the work that we do.

It seems that some health care professionals particularly enjoy 'making people better', in the sense that they recover from their illness or that their debility improves. They may choose to work in areas where end-of-life care is less prevalent (Mackintosh 2007), and the principal ethos of the work will be one of curing disease. Professional caring in this way is clearly hugely valuable work. When care has focused on curing disease or improving debility but nevertheless the patient dies, rather than feeling good because we have helped someone, health care professionals can feel a sense of failure. Death in such circumstances confronts us with the limitations of health care and the fragility that life holds.

The focus of Mark's care was rehabilitation. Rehabilitation aims to improve patients' quality of life, often through maximising independence in the context of illness and disability. Rehabilitation is generally associated with long-term illness and disability in which a steady improvement or adaptation can be expected (National Council for Hospice and Specialist Palliative Care Services 2000). In the case of Mark, sadly that expectation was unfulfilled.

Thinking about Peter, it is likely that he found a strong desire to care, possibly influenced by unexpectedly becoming his sick wife's carer. He may have particularly enjoyed the sense of fulfilment that caring can bring. He may also have particularly enjoyed caring for Mark as they had shared interests. However, Mark's untimely death may have confronted Peter with loss and sadness which possibly resonated with his own bereavement.

How I might be affected when a patient dies

Like many students, Peter kept a reflective diary. The following excerpt from it illustrates some of the common thoughts and feelings that students experience following the death of a patient they have cared for.

Peter's diary

At last it's over. A dreadful shift. I was even looking forward to going back to the rehab ward this morning. It has been a good placement up till today, really nice patients many of them quite young and a good laugh to be with. It was nice looking after Mark as we could talk bikes. He really seemed to appreciate me being around. To find he had just died out of the blue was gutting. Why couldn't the doctors have done something to stop the bleeding? I don't get it. Last week I said I would bring in a picture of my old Triumph but I had forgotten until today. I feel really guilty about that.

Sally, my mentor, asked me if I wanted to carry out last offices. We had covered this in the skills lab at uni but I was really nervous. Looking back, that uni session just hadn't prepared me for what to expect at all. Mark looked just awful, so drained somehow. He was quite warm underneath which was a bit eerie. Sally was weird too. She kept talking to him all the way though just like doing a bed bath. Why on earth did she do that? The worst bit was when we dressed him in a disposable shroud thing, then wrapped in a sheet, put him in a body bag and then labels.... He just wasn't Mark anymore. Covering the face was awful – I started to well up at that bit.

Sally and I went on break afterwards and she asked me how I was. I know she was trying to be supportive and in a way she was, but she seemed so normal as if it was an everyday thing to her. I will never see it like that.

Later, after lunch, Sue (Mark's wife) came on to the ward and made a beeline for me. I think she had been to the relative's officer or something. I did not know her very well but she looked awful. She just said thank you for chatting with Mark, he enjoyed it. I just said 'That's OK'. I didn't know what else to say to her. I could have told her about Lyn, my wife maybe. Sally sent me home after that.

Although students are affected by the death of a patient in many different ways, Peter's diary excerpt shows a number of common responses, including shock, confusion, guilt and anger. These feelings are all identified within research in the field.

Parry (2011) explored student nurses' first experience of death in clinical practice through a focus group of five students. Like Peter, these students found the experience traumatic and were shocked by the appearance of the dead body. Clearly, feeling shocked by death is very common. Wrapping the body is emotionally very difficult. Cooper and Barnett (2005) suggest this is because it is the point at which a patient starts to be treated differently from someone who is unconscious, thus transforming them into a corpse. Parry (2011) found that many students found classroom teaching of limited value in preparing them for patients' deaths, so that in practice the experience still comes as a shock.

Action point

It is common to feel shocked by the death of a patient and particularly by their appearance after death. Most people in contemporary Britain do not have direct experience of death (see Chapter 1 for more discussion about this). Do not expect that you will be unaffected by it. This is not unprofessional in any sense. Do talk about your feelings with your mentor and tutors. Although they might manage their emotions differently, sharing your reaction with them can be helpful.

Peter's feeling of guilt that he had not been able to show Mark the picture as he had promised is also understandable. Cooper and Barnett's (2005) exploration of first-year student nurses' experiences of death found that they felt guilty when unexpected death prevented the 'extra special care' that students wished to give dying patients.

Action point

After someone has died, it is common to feel guilty and wish that we had done things differently. Try to remember the positive care you gave in circumstances where there were many other demands on your time. In the main, patients and families value the sense of caring that is conveyed by professionals. Despite Peter forgetting to bring the picture, he clearly cared about Mark and Sue appreciated that.

Peter's feelings of anger at Mark's death, and that doctors did not prevent it, are also understandable. It can seem incomprehensible that death has occurred despite all that modern medical care can offer. Anger is a common response to loss and is described in many bereavement models (Kübler-Ross 1969; Parkes 1986). While these models are based on the experiences of patients and relatives, they involve common emotions that people experience following loss. They are therefore transferable to other situations. While Peter's feelings of anger towards Mark's doctors may be understandable, it is important to appreciate that it is unreasonable.

Action point

If you feel anger at colleagues following the death of a patient, wait until it subsides. Talking it over with a friend or peer or writing it down can help.

Consider calmly whether it is reasonable. You may discuss the situation with a mentor or tutor. There may be an explanation. Remember that your colleagues may also be affected by his unexpected death and have a host of feelings associated with it. While anger is understandable, avoid allowing it to hurt colleagues.

Peter is not alone in finding speaking to relatives after a death upsetting to the point of wanting to cry. Clearly the situation is immensely sad and this is a very reasonable reaction. Relatives may well be comforted by students crying, as it shows that their loved one had been cared for by someone who was touched by their life. However, be careful that your distress does not overwhelm the relative, putting them in a situation where they feel concern for your welfare. This might add to their already considerable emotional burden.

A couple of weeks later Peter writes again in his journal ...

CASE STUDY

Peter's diary

I am still bothered by Mark's sudden death and am beginning to feel down about it. I thought I had got over how Jan [Peter's wife] died but now I am not so sure. I can't believe that you can be alive and kicking one minute and dead the next. I thought nursing was supposed to be about helping people. I am now not sure what the point is.

I've talked to Gemma about it a bit but I don't like to say too much to her about Jan. Sally just seems to have forgotten about it now. How on earth do you just 'get used to it'? I don't know what to do.

In Parry's (2011) focus group, described earlier in this chapter, all of the students wanted to talk to someone other than their mentor about their experience after the death of a patient (Parry 2011). It seems that caring for a patient who dies can trigger thoughts and emotions relating to personal experiences, as the second extract from Peter's reflective diary shows. Terry and Carroll (2008) found that this can become very traumatic for some, with evidence in their study of students having flashbacks of dying patients, and subsequently developing techniques to distance themselves from the impact of caring for dead patients. Clearly, for some, the death of a patient can be hugely challenging, leading to a rethink of their career choices. It may also be isolating and depressing.

> ## Action point
>
> There is no right or wrong way to be affected by a patient's death. However, it is helpful to develop an awareness of how and to what extent you are affected, not only by the death of a patient, but also by any other aspect of care. Appreciating the challenge you face is important so that you can assess the support you need.

> ## Example from the author's experience
>
> I was 22 when I qualified as a nurse and, at 23, nursed patients with Acquired Human Immunodeficiency Virus (AIDS) at a time when they commonly died some months after diagnosis. I found the death of patients who were younger than me to be particularly distressing. I was looking forward to my adult life and found it hugely poignant that their whole lives were shorter than mine had been so far. I found it helpful to bring this to a support group held for staff on the ward. I found that others shared my reaction.

How registered practitioners might be affected by patients' deaths

It is not uncommon to feel shocked that qualified practitioners appear simply to carry on to the next task as the dead patient's bed is quickly taken by someone else (Parry 2011). While this approach can seem uncaring, it is more likely that it masks the deeper impact that caring for dying patients can have.

Research by McCloskey and Taggart (2010) sheds light on the impact that caring for children can have on one group of health professionals – children's paediatric nurses. They analysed four focus groups: one group comprised children's nurses working in a hospice, two groups were comprised of community children's nurses and the fourth group was of specialist hospital-based children's nurses. The research found that competing and overpowering demands were a considerable source of stress for these nurses. Some felt more worn down by the accumulation of sadness they had encountered with the many patients and families they had cared for over time, rather than by their contacts with specific individuals to whom they had become particularly attached. Some cited the burden of time and resource constraints limiting the quality of care that they were able to deliver; others raised the challenges of both living and working in the same community as sources of stress. The research highlighted that the relationship between sick patients and nurses was both satisfying and emotionally stressful as the nurses became increasingly aware of the difficulties and loss in patients' lives. In addition, the limited control that nurses can have over the events and environment around them emerged as challenging. Like Mark, many patients face uncertain times, making care needs unpredictable. This lack of certainty can be very stressful.

The research gives useful insight into the pressures on qualified nurses. Qualified nurses are affected by the death of a patient, but perhaps in a different way from students. Remember that other professional groups are also affected. Occupational therapists, physiotherapists, doctors and dieticians were all involved in Mark's care, and may well have been shocked by his death. Similarly, ancillary staff such as cleaners, porters and clerical staff may have felt shocked.

It is important to avoid stereotypes and judgements about who may or may not be emotionally affected by Mark's death, as it cuts through professional boundaries and roles. Remember that different people may express their sadness differently and often more experienced staff may simply carry on; but it does not mean that they do not care or are not affected.

The sources of support that are available

Support systems that mitigate the emotional impact that caring for dying patients may have are important (McCloskey and Taggart 2010). Accessing support relies on recognising the way you respond to challenging situations and what helps you to manage your response in a positive way. For example, this may be as simple as recognising that you have cared for a lot of people facing loss this week and you are feeling low, so it is important to balance that with doing something fun on your days off. Or, if one patient is really troubling you, it might be helpful to make some time to talk to your mentor about it.

People vary in the type of support that they have and how they use it. For many, having supportive friends, colleagues and family, with whom they can enjoy leisure time and possibly discuss concerns, is the foundation of the support network they have. Sharing hard times as a health care team by simply chatting in a coffee break or having a night out together can be a great support. It can be very helpful to balance the sadness you witness in patients' lives with having fun, being physically active and enjoying interests outside work. For some, faith and spiritual beliefs can be a huge source of personal support.

Sources of professional support offered in practice may include reflective practice sessions, clinical supervision and informal access to colleagues and managers in order to discuss concerns. Employers (such as hospitals) often offer access to occupational counselling services if needed.

For students, mentors are an obvious place to turn. Universities offer personal tutors, practice educators and clinical teachers who are all likely to be able to offer support. Sometimes the process of reflecting through essays and diaries such as Peter's journal can be helpful. Many universities have specific well-being services, such as student counselling services.

If the burden of caring weighs heavily or for some time, it may be appropriate to seek help from your general practitioner (GP). Mark's death has significantly upset Peter, perhaps raising the issue of the cost that emotional attachment can bring, and also bringing back the grief Peter felt on his wife's death. In this circumstance he could well be helped by bereavement counselling.

Reflective question

Which support mechanisms might be helpful to you in managing your own feelings following the death of patients?

Different people find different ways of managing their own feelings following a death of a patient. Many may enjoy social time with their colleagues – a good night out. Others seek support from peers or friends and family, with whom they can share their experiences. Try to develop an awareness of what is difficult for you and what will support you.

Burnout

'Burnout' describes fatigue that affects caring professionals. It is characterised by emotional exhaustion, in which a person feels unable to give any more of their emotional self. This creates a sense of depersonalisation, whereby practitioners become cold and distant to colleagues as well as to patients. This can make them appear callous. It can also affect their ability to follow things through to completion, manifesting as an 'it doesn't really matter' approach, in which they can seem fatalistic and incompetent (Pereira et al. 2011).

Burnout can be viewed as a response to cumulative difficult experiences in caring. It is unlikely that students will experience it directly. It is more likely that you will meet practitioners who are suffering from it later in their careers. In their systematic review of burnout in palliative care, Pereira et al. (2011) found that lack of confidence in communication skills, pressures of time and dealing with pain, suffering and dying, were all risk factors in developing burnout. The reality of burnout challenges us not only to look after ourselves, but also to be considerate and caring of colleagues. We need to note and offer support to others who are emotionally affected by caring work.

Developing resilience

Resilience describes the human trait that enables people to endure and overcome the effects of difficulties (Newman and Blackburn 2002). For example, Nelson Mandela can be described as hugely resilient since he retained his personal integrity and leadership ability despite years of imprisonment. The concept of resilience is interesting, since developing it may help health care practitioners resolve feelings of sadness following the death of a patient.

Being resilient to the effects of caring for dying patients does not mean losing the compassion that motivates us to care and that patients and families greatly appreciate. It does not necessarily mean not experiencing sadness when a patient has died. Rather, it involves finding ways to continue to care for people who are experiencing huge loss despite the sadness that we may inevitably experience.

Many of the studies undertaken on resilience have considered why particular children from disadvantaged circumstances have fared considerably better than the majority of their peers. Monroe and Oliviere (2006) wonder whether the factors which seem to promote resilience in these children can also be used to help us find ways to manage our own feelings of sadness when someone has died.

One such factor cited by Monroe and Oliviere (2006) is the ability to identify positive aspects of hardship. For example, this might be that a missed holiday, while sad, also enabled time to be spent at home with friends. When applying this to Peter's case, recognising the value of the relationship Peter gave to Mark may mitigate Peter's feeling of sadness at his death.

In addition, Monroe and Oliviere (2006) highlight the significance of social support networks in enabling children to develop resilience.

Returning to Peter's case

Hopefully, with good support Peter may come to feel more positively about his caring experience with Mark. Mark's death was beyond anyone's control and while sad, comfort may be taken from the fact that he had been well cared for and that Peter had significantly improved Mark's enjoyment of life in his last weeks and days. For Peter, the knowledge of this may mitigate his feelings of despondency so that his chosen career may be fulfilling.

Summary

The key points to remember when resolving our own feeling when a patient dies are:

- It is important to be aware of what made and makes you want to be a professional carer, what challenges you emotionally and what support helps you.
- Being upset by the death of a patient is common and OK!
- Consider that others, including more senior staff, are also challenged by caring work, but may show this very differently. They may need you in turn to notice and support them.
- Try to foster your own emotional resilience to manage the emotional impact of caring work.

Further reading

Smith, P. (2012) *The Emotional Labour of Nursing Revisited: Can Nurses Still Care?* Basingstoke: Palgrave Macmillan. This book explores the impact that caring in contemporary health care has on nurses. In particular, it includes consideration of the impact of caring for dying patients.

Howatson-Jones, L. (2010) *Reflective Practice in Nursing*. Exeter: Learning Matters. This book is one of a number of good guides to reflective practice in nursing.

References

Cooper, J. and Barnett, M. (2005) 'Aspects of caring for dying patients which cause anxiety to first-year student nurses', *International Journal of Palliative Nursing*, 11(8): 423–30.

Kirby, C. (2003) 'Commitment to care: a philosophical perspective on nursing', Chapter 2 in L. Basford and O. Slevin (eds), *Theory and Practice of Nursing* (2nd edn). Cheltenham: Nelson Thornes.

Kübler-Ross, E. (1969) *On Death and Dying*. London and New York: Routledge.

Mackintosh, C. (2007) 'Making patients better: a qualitative descriptive study of registered nurses' reasons for working in surgical areas', *Journal of Clinical Nursing*, 16(6): 1134–40.

McCloskey S. and Taggart, L. (2010) 'How much compassion have I left? An exploration of occupational stress among children's palliative care nurses', *International Journal of Palliative Nursing*, 16(5): 233–40.

Monroe, B. and Oliviere, D. (2006) 'Resilience in palliative care', *European Journal of Palliative Care*, 13(1): 22–5.

National Council for Hospice and Specialist Palliative Care Services (August 2000) 'Fulfilling lives: rehabilitation in palliative care'. London: National Council for Hospice and Specialist Palliative Care Services.

Newman, T. and Blackburn, S. (2002) *Transitions in the Lives of Children and Young People: Resilience Factors – Summary* (Interchange 78). Edinburgh: Scottish Education Department.

Newton, J.M., Kelly, C.M., Kremser, A.K., Jolly, B. and Billett, S. (2009) 'The motivations to nurse: an exploration of factors amongst undergraduate students, registered nurses and nurse managers', *Journal of Nursing Management*, 17(3): 392–400.

Parkes, C.M. (1986) *Bereavement*. Harmondsworth: Penguin.

Parry, M. (2011) 'Student nurses' experience of their first death in clinical practice', *International Journal of Palliative Nursing*, 17(9): 448–53.

Pereira, S., Fonseca, A. and Carvalho, A. (2011) 'Burnout in palliative care: a systematic review', *Nursing Ethics*, 18(3): 317–26.

Terry, L.M. and Carroll, J. (2008) 'Dealing with death: first encounters for first-year nursing students', *British Journal of Nursing*, 17(12): 760–5.

Author index

Subject index